# Smart Guide™

## to

# Sports Medicine

Sheila Sobell

CADER BOOKS

**John Wiley & Sons, Inc.**

New York • Chichester • Weinheim • Brisbane • Singapore • Toronto

*Library of Congress Cataloging-in-Publication Data:*
Sobell, Sheila.
Smart guide to sports medicine / Sheila Sobell.
p.        cm.
Includes index.
ISBN 0-471-35647-6 (pbk.)
1. Sports medicine; popular works.  I. Title.
RC1210.S623                    1999
617.1'027—dc21                99-27222

Printed in the United States of America

10  9  8  7  6  5  4  3  2  1

*To Richard Nicholas Every,*
*muse, cheerleader, researcher,*
*friend and inspiration*

# Acknowledgments

Grateful acknowedgment is made to the following individuals and institutions:

Dorothy Beach of the American Society of Journalists and authors, for opening doors.
Richard Every and Steve Moramarco for invaluable research.
Ellen and John Every for fact checking.
The American Podiatric Medical Association.
The American Orthopaedic Foot and Ankle Society.
The Penn State Sports Newsletter.
The Sporting Goods Manufacturers Association.
The American Orthopaedic Society for Sports Medicine.
The American Council on Exercise.
The American Dietetic Association.
Karen Freeman M.S. R.D., University of California, San Diego School of Medicine.
Lee Rice, D.O., San Diego Sports Medicine Center, Inc.
University of California, San Diego, School of Medicine.
Denise Wiksten, Ph.D., A.T.C., San Diego State University.
Gene Lemke, Ph.D., San Diego State University.
Peter Francis, Ph.D., San Diego State University.
Georgia Tech Sports Medicine & Performance Newsletter.
The American Chiropractic Association.
Dave Yukelson, Ph.D., Penn State University.
American Academy of Orthopaedic Surgeons.

# Contents

# Introduction

In 1995, my new husband and I had a wild and crazy idea—to pursue a dream we'd both secretly had of spending idle days sailing the Mediterranean. We bought a small 20-year old English catamaran and embarked on an 18-month odyssey that took us from Turkey through the Greek isles, southern Italy, and the canals of France en route to Britain. Nothing about the voyage proved idle apart from its initial conception; as the result of a force-10 gale and the physical rigors of the sporting life at sea, between us we injured almost every anatomical structure on our left sides (in addition to my coccyx).

Having returned to the States both with a bad case of "left" and the unusual distinction of having mastered the way to describe a variety of sports injuries in several foreign languages, I come to the writing of this book with considerable personal experience. the Smart Guide to Sports Medicine starts by examining the benefits of the sporting life and what would-be athletes need to know to get the most out of it safely. Whether you're just getting into sports, adding something new, or trying to get those aging muscles back into shape, chapter 1 will map out conditioning and training programs designed to make your body as able as your spirit is willing. You'll also discover the profile of the athlete at risk for injury and the most common mistakes that send budding athletes to the sidelines. You'll get the latest scoop on what to eat to power your play, the equipment to make your moves swift and deft, and how to develop the mental attitude to give you that competitive edge.

The remainder of the book deals with a subject I mastered firsthand at sea—pain and its relationship to sports. You'll learn that it's often our misconceptions about pain that gets us into trouble. For example, we gain nothing—other than upping our risk for an overuse injury—by pushing through pain. You'll also discover how to differentiate between minor and major injuries, how to treat them, and when it's safe to resume play. The goals are to prevent minor injuries from escalating in seriousness and to harness the healing power of the mind.

The next several chapters tackle the issues of injury prevention, diagnosis, treatment, and rehabilitation as we examine what can go wrong when we hit the sports playing field. The information is organized anatomically from head to toe, so it's easy to find and even easier to implement.

In the sport-by-sport guide, you'll learn what types of injuries are most prevalent and the precautions necessary to keep you safe. If you do get hurt, you'll have a no-nonsense guide to diagnosing the injury and determining whether it needs first aid or the healing skills of a physician.

Women have special needs long ignored by the manufacturers of sports equipment. In chapter 7, we'll consider just how anatomy is destiny, what sports are appropriate during pregnancy, how to buy a sports bra, and how to avoid certain injuries for which female athletes are at risk. Middle-aged and older people will learn how to safely condition their bodies so that getting back into the game at any age can be remarkably rewarding and safe.

The final chapter describes breakthroughs in treating orthopedic injuries. Scientists actually now know how to grow new bone to mend hard-to-heal bone fractures, use radio-frequency heat probes to shrink overstretched tendons, administer quick relief to the point of pain via a pain patch, and much, much more. Whether you, like I, have a bad case of "left," a knee that's given out from too much running on hard surfaces, or a tennis elbow that suffers reinjury, advances in sports medicine can literally and figuratively make a new athlete of you.

# CHAPTER 1

......................

# On Your Mark!

Congratulations! So you've just cleaned out your closet and found your old tennis racquet and spent the afternoon reminiscing over your glory days as a high school tennis star. Maybe now's the time to shape up those middle-aged muscles and find out if you still have what it takes on the courts. Or maybe that persistent pain in your elbow has finally persuaded you to exchange your golf clubs for a bicycle.

Whether you're getting into sports for the first time or adding a new sport to your repertoire, the physical and psychological returns on your effort will be substantial. Employing a sensible plan and suitable equipment, plus guidance from coaches, trainers, and more experienced players, is the smart way to ensure your enthusiasm will be matched by improved physical conditioning and a mastery of new skills essential to the game.

# The Benefits of a Sporting Life

Whether your recreational sport of choice is aerobic dancing, running, squash, cycling, or skating, the positive impact of the sporting life on overall health is indisputable. For women, weight-bearing exercises like these have a dramatic effect on reducing the risk of osteoporosis by slowing the rate of bone loss while improving muscle tone in arteries and veins, cutting the risk of heart attack and stroke.

Though there have been few studies on the impact of engaging in specific sports on overall health, an enormous body of scientific research does link physical activity (the key element in sport) with increased longevity and reduced risk of disease.

The Department of Kinesiology Health at Georgia State University has said that being physically active reduces the risks of premature death, developing and/or dying from heart disease, and developing certain cancers and diabetes.

At the same time, physical activity builds and maintains healthy muscles, bones, and joints and improves psychological well-being. Regular participation in sports ups the zest factor, reducing depression and anxiety while improving mood. And because being around someone with a positive mental attitude is fun, happier people have more friends.

The more and the harder you play, the greater the benefits, says Paul Williams of the Berkeley National Laboratory, key researcher on a National Runner's Health Study comparing the health effects of vigorous and moderate running on women's health. The findings showed that vigorous play pays off with a significant increase in HDL levels (the "good" cholesterol) beyond what's achieved in moderate running.

# Evaluating Your Baseline Fitness

Before lacing up your shoes and hitting the courts, it's a smart idea to have a baseline fitness evaluation to examine your overall strength, flexibility, and endurance—the key elements involved in playing sports. That way you'll know what type of conditioning program will maximize your ability to play well and without injury.

Both athletic and personal trainers are certified to perform a baseline fitness evaluation, which is usually done at minimal cost. A standard evaluation generally consists of four parts—steps, sit and reach, push-ups, and sit-ups. Scores in each area are rated from "Very Poor" to "Superior," based on tables comparing your performance with others of your gender and age.

• Stepping up and down off a box for three minutes measures cardiovascular conditioning.

• The sit-and-reach test measures hamstring flexibility—how far toward your toes you can reach while sitting on the floor with legs extended and knees locked.

• Both the push-up (measuring overall strength and muscular endurance) and the sit-up (gauging abdominal strength) tests are performed against the clock. Scoring is based on the number of repetitions completed in one minute.

"Once we've established your baseline fitness, the next step is to develop a conditioning program to build overall strength, flexibility, and endurance specific to the sport you want to play," says Nick Holslag, a certified personal trainer (CPT) at Renaissance Personal Training in San Diego.

For more conditioned athletes interested in pursuing new sports interests, bench presses to evaluate upper body strength and the Roman chair to measure lower back strength are usually added.

# Getting a Clean Bill of Health

Before starting an exercise plan, see your doctor for a physical if you have chronic diseases such as heart disease or diabetes, or if you're at high risk for developing these diseases. Also check with your doctor if you have frequent dizzy spells; extreme breathlessness after mild exertion; arthritis (or bone problems); or severe muscular, ligament, or tendon problems. Men over age 40 and women over age 50 should also consult with their doctors.

We've all heard scare stories about people seemingly in the best of health who suffer an unexpected heart attack playing sports. That's more myth than fact. Even though the odds of a myocardial infarction among people who are regularly active elevates somewhat during physical exertion, the risk is actually less than for those who are sedentary. Though rare, serious exercise-related medical emergencies occur primarily among those who are sedentary, have advanced arteriosclerotic disease (thickening and loss of elasticity of the artery walls), and who undertook strenuous exertion without proper conditioning.

# Choosing the Best Sport for Your Body

Although your vulnerabilities shouldn't keep you out of the game, they should be considered when deciding which sport to play.

## SMART SOURCES

The following organizations can help you find a sports medicine professional to assist with a fitness evaluation:

The National Athletic
    Trainer's Association
2952 Stremmons
    Freeway
Dallas, TX 75247-
    6916
(214) 637-6282
www.nata.org

National Federation of
    Professional Trainers
(800) 729-6378
www.nfpt.com

The American College
    of Sports Medicine
    (ACSM)
PO Box 1440
Indianapolis, IN
    46206-1440
(317) 637-9200
www.sportsmed.org

With over 17,000 members, ACSM is the largest organization of sports and medicine professionals. Their web site lists member physicians according to city and zip code.

Occasional aches and pains like sore shoulders, backache, or knee pains are no excuse to rule out playing sports. "The safest thing to do is to listen to your body," says Dr. Nick DiNubble, an orthopedic surgeon who contributed to the *Surgeon General's Report on Physical Activity and Health.* "If something hurts, modify your sports program, but don't let it force you out of the game. In most cases, exercise is the best prescription for reducing or even eliminating pain, especially if you have conditions like arthritis or low back pain."

• **Aching Knees.** Running isn't the best choice for those with knee pain. But cycling actually helps rehabilitate the knee joint. Building the strength of thigh muscles and increasing hamstring flexibility will also help alleviate pain.

• **Shoulder Pain.** Shoulder pain generally indicates overuse of the joint. Stretch your shoulders thoroughly before playing. Strengthening the rotator cuff muscle supporting the shoulder should help you feel strong enough to play tennis or swim. Just don't overdo it.

• **Low Back Pain.** Sports like golf, skiing, and tennis that involve considerable bending and twisting aren't advised if you have frequent bouts of backache. But swimming, coupled with exercises to strengthen back muscles, can help you feel good enough to play other sports.

# Implementing Universal Training Principles

How do you get from the starting position to the finish line without becoming injured? Suppose your goal is to be able to play tennis for an hour. But if you've been lax about exercising, your aerobic fitness is probably at Love.

## 1. Concentrate on Duration, Frequency, and Intensity

To become really competent at sports, you need to improve how long, how frequently, and how hard you play. That's accomplished by increasing one variable at at time by 10 percent until you've attained your performance goals. *Caution:* Never alter more than one variable at a time; doing so puts you at risk for a stress injury!

Here are a few sport-specific examples for working on these variables:

### Jogging

Start with about 20 minutes of combined walking and jogging three times a week. Go at a moderate pace that allows you to converse comfortably. Increase the frequency of the workout by 10 percent a week until you're walking/running four or five days. Then increase duration 10 percent a week until you reach goal. Finally, increase intensity by adding hills or small bursts of explosive speed.

### Golf

What counts in golf is your total number of swings. To develop swings that are consistent in movement and speed from the 1st to the 18th hole, start by hitting balls on the driving range. Monitor your level of soreness. While some is to be expected, soreness shouldn't interfere with normal movement patterns and should disappear with repeated activity. Then increase playtime 10 percent so that you're on the range longer and hitting more balls. Finally, train for intensity by varying terrain and position. For example, play on a slant with one leg up or try to drive the ball out of a trap.

### Racquet Sports

Get technique, rhythm, balance, and shot selection down by hitting some balls against the backboard. To learn how to position yourself to serve and receive, add a partner. Start off playing for 20 minutes, adding 10 percent more each week until

## SMART MOVE

"To prevent injuries, start out with what seems at first a ridiculously easy amount of exertion," says Lee Rice, D.O., medical director of the Sports Medicine Center in San Diego. "Then make sure your body can handle the same amount of exertion on several different occasions. As soon as you feel you're doing more than you can comfortably handle, back off. The goal of training is to 'overload' muscles with small incremental increases in workload, making muscle fibers stronger. Soon you'll have the endurance to run for 30 minutes or play 9 holes of golf."

the duration of play is where you want it. Next, increase intensity for the middle 15 minutes by striving harder for out-of-range balls. Use more explosive force. Then, resume practice, gradually cooling down.

## 2. Strengthen and Tone Muscles

Like the heart, muscles must be conditioned for strength and endurance. For a strong lower back and midsection—requirements in most sports—pelvic tilts, sit-ups and abdominal crunches are recommended. Technique counts. Don't do sit-ups with feet hooked under a chair; otherwise, your hip flexor muscles will work harder than your abs. Instead, begin with bent-knee crunches in which knees are bent and feet planted squarely on the floor. Lift your head and shoulders, holding for about three seconds. Gradually progress to arms across chest; then behind your head.

To smash a tennis ball over the net or go the distance swimming, you'll need strength. Every would-be sports player should weight train twice a week for 20 minutes, working all the major muscle groups. Otherwise, the muscle density you had in your twenties will decline as you age. Rest 48 hours between workouts. Weight training actually produces tiny muscle tears that temporarily decrease strength and increase soreness.

## 3. Stretching for Flexibility

For the suppleness to hit a long shot two hundred yards onto the fairway, you need a sport-specific stretching program that will ensure a full range of motion. Golfers, for example, should loosen shoulders and upper back muscles; racquet players need to stretch their thighs and calves. In studies on the effect of stretching, Brigham Young University and Louisiana State University researchers found that static stretching (holding a stretch without bouncing) improved performance in sports requiring strength and power.

## 4. Condition Your Heart

When engaging in aerobic sports like jogging and racquet sports, which work your heart and cardiovascular system, aim for your target heart rate. This represents the rate that best conditions and strengthens the heart so it can pump blood most efficiently.

# Sport-Specific Training

Although the ability to play any sport depends on your aerobic capacity, strength, and flexibility, each sport puts unique demands on specific muscle groups. To ensure that your body is up to the challenge, consult with a coach or trainer to develop sport-specific toning and stretching exercises. Concentrating on these areas will increase blood flow to ligaments, tendons, and muscles so that they respond more easily and safely.

Here are training recommendations for some of the more popular sport activities.

### Skiing
Strengthen thighs and calves with exercises like squat exchanges and pillow jumps (leaping over a pillow sideways with both feet). And don't forget stretches for calves.

**F.Y.I.**

To determine target heart rate, use the following formula:

1. Calculate your maximum heart rate (the greatest number of times your heart can safely beat per minute during exercise) by subtracting your age from 220.

2. Multiply by 70%.

*Thus:*
[220 – age] × 70% = Target heart rate

Example: Target heart rate for a 40-year-old:
220 – 40 = 180
180 × .70 = 126
Target heart rate is 126 heart beats per minute.

### Golf

Weight train to strengthen biceps to generate sufficient club head speed for hitting the ball long distances. Weight train with machines designed to increase range of motion in trunk. Incorporate strengthening and flexibility exercise for hamstrings and legs.

### Running

Stretch as often as four times daily, concentrating on the groin, hamstrings, and calves.

### Cycling

Weight train to strengthen trunk and legs. Stretch trunk, thighs, calves, and hamstrings.

### In-line Skating

Weight train to strengthen hip muscles for side-to-side movement. Stretch trunk, hip flexor muscles, hamstrings, and calves.

### Racquet Sports

Weight train for arms and upper back. Add rotational exercises for hips. Stretch upper and lower legs and hamstrings.

### Swimming

Stretch shoulders and hips.

# Profile of the Athlete at Risk for Injury

Lots of variables—faulty equipment, poorly maintained playing surfaces, or fatigue—can cause an athlete to become injured. Probably the most important—your mental outlook—is something you can control. A slight attitude adjustment can make the difference between being injury- or safety-prone. What's the profile of the athlete most likely to get hurt?

## The Weekend Warrior

You've seen them yourselves—weekend athletes hot to hit the court with everything they've got. Never mind that they do zero conditioning Monday through Friday; they'll make up for it on the weekend. Warriors come in all sizes and genders—what they have in common is the tendency to ask their bodies to do more than they can.

## The Would-Be Athlete on a Mission

Overweight, overworked, but not necessarily competitive, these would-be athletes have taken New Year's resolutions to the max. So what if they've done nothing for the last 32 months but consider the bottom line on the spreadsheet at the expense of their own spreading bottoms. Lesser men than they have run a four-minute mile, so can they . . .

## Type A's

So competitive they'll play through pain, thinking it's good for them. As likely to be injured fighting as they are playing, they'll get into it over a wrong call or a bad play.

## The Greatly Stressed

On stress overload and looking for relief, these types suffer from anxiety-induced muscle tension, which leads to muscle guarding, decreased flexi-

**SMART MOVE**

"Many adults still think they're kids and treat their bodies as if they still were," says Gene Lemke, Ph.D., professor of recreation, parks, and tourism at San Diego State University. "Because they're living in the past, they work their bodies the same way they did when they were twenty. So they go out and skate for an afternoon, forgetting to build up their endurance and flexibility slowly. Invariably, they develop a stress fracture, and the skates wind up back in the closet!"

bility, and impaired motor coordination. If they can't turn off the office, their inability to give the game their full attention will lead to tight muscles and poor concentration—and injury.

# Avoiding Common Athletic Mistakes

Now that you have a clear understanding of how attitude affects the possibility of injury, the next step is to analyze your performance habits, weeding out those that may undermine the joy of playing safely and well.

• **Take Your Time.** "The classic example of someone who does too much too soon are skiers who want to make up for the fact that it's a seasonal sport," says Lee Rice. "They're ready mentally to pick up where they left off last winter. Unfortunately, their bodies aren't. Instead of taking a bit of time to get back in the groove of things, they push themselves to ski all day on the most advanced runs."

• **Change One Variable at a Time.** Becoming conditioned is a gradual process in which frequency, duration, and intensity are increased one at a time at a progression of 10 percent per week until performance goals are reached.

• **Rest When Fatigued.** Stop playing when you're tired. Fatigue affects concentration, coordination, endurance, speed, judgment, and alertness, any and all of which compromise safety.

• **Correct Biomechanical Faults.** Begin a new sport with know-how from a pro. That's the smart way to avoid developing biomechanical faults like running with an awkward or asymmetrical gait, throwing in a way that stresses the elbow, or adopting an incorrect posture that can hinder performance and cause injuries.

• **Choose Sport-Friendly Surfaces.** Opt for well-maintained surfaces and terrain that will keep you and other athletes in a position to compete safely. Beware of situations that almost invariably lead to injuries, like running downhill on concrete or playing tennis on poorly maintained surfaces.

• **Pay Attention to Overuse Symptoms.** Listen to your body so that you can stop playing when pain becomes sharper. Watch for swelling and stiffness in joints. Take time out if pain increases with just minor movement.

• **Take Time to Recover.** Protect against overuse injuries by taking time between playing for your body to recover and adapt to progressive increases in workloads.

• **Include Warm-Ups and Cooldowns.** Muscles, ligaments, and tendons require proper conditioning to avoid strains and tears. To head-off stiffness, begin and end your activity with stretches. To rev metabolism and improve muscle elasticity, start by exercising in slow motion the muscle groups you'll use. For example, runners should walk-jog slowly, increasing to a run. Swimmers should do a few laps, and racquet players rally with a partner. This also readies your heart for aerobic exertion. Once the heart and muscle temperature is warmed,

## STREET SMARTS

Jane Every, a 36-year-old public relations consultant, was late for her aerobic dancing class. The instructor had finished the last of the stretches in the warm-up. Jane was at a critical juncture. "I'd been warned over and over how important it was to warm up," she admits. "If I'd been smart, I would have skipped the class and worked out on the weights. But I thought I could get away without it since I swam a lot."

When her back went out because she wasn't warmed up, Jane endured weeks of acupuncture to get the pain under control.

"I learned the facts of sport fitness the hard way," she admits. "The cardinal rule of warming up your muscles before you exercise them is true. If I'd done what I knew was smart, I wouldn't have messed up my back."

**SMART MOVE**

"To stay focused on what you want to occur, rather than on mistakes, learn to develop a mental plan," advises Dave Yukelson, Ph.D., sports psychologist at Penn State's Morgan Academic Support Center for Student Athletes. "For example, if you're playing tennis, concentrate on what you have to do to beat your opponent; how to force him to make errors; how to be ready to move when he does. Visualize your goal, and play fully focused with complete confidence."

slowly stretch your muscles to increase their ability to respond to the demands of playing. Post game, give your heart a break by cooling down gradually instead of stopping suddenly.

# Psych Up to Play

Any time you play against an opponent, you'll confront the occasional bad break like a missed shot or unfair call. How you handle disappointment just may give you the winning edge.

If the inevitable happens, and you blow it, learn to let go. "All of us make mistakes," says Dave Yukelson, Ph.D., sports psychologist at Penn State's Morgan Academic Support Center for Student Athletes. "The trick is not to allow one mistake to spiral down into another. Refocus your mental attitude and your technique. Suppose it's 'four all' and your doubles buddy hits an easy ball wide into the net. You can choose to throw an attitude muscle and play the rest of the game tight and frustrated. Or you can decide to play one point at a time and stay centered with the right thoughts."

Learning to deal with adversity is key to making the game enjoyable. "Develop a pre-performance routine, and visualize ahead of time how you'll react when things go wrong," Yukelson says. "Acknowledge that you made a horrible mistake, take a deep breath, let go of anger. Then relax and move into the ball, concentrating on what you have to do to get back to deuce."

In the end, it's how you respond to mistakes and refocus your concentration that leads to wins and good self-esteem.

# Myths and Facts about Nutrition

Athletes often have many misconceptions about sports nutrition. They assume that carbohydrates come in only one form—starch. Following the advice that 60 percent of an athlete's diet should come from carbohydrates, they eat too much bread, pasta, and rice, neglecting other sources like dairy, fruits, and vegetables essential to a balanced diet.

Since Americans have been urged to restrict intake of both red meat and fat, many would-be athletes think they can go one better by eliminating fat completely. That means they may not consume enough calories to manufacture glycogen needed for muscle energy.

The basis for a sound eating plan is the Food Guide Pyramid.

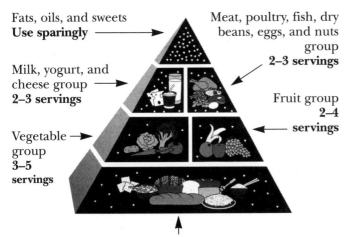

Fats, oils, and sweets
**Use sparingly**

Meat, poultry, fish, dry beans, eggs, and nuts group
**2–3 servings**

Milk, yogurt, and cheese group
**2–3 servings**

Fruit group
**2–4 servings**

Vegetable group
**3–5 servings**

Bread, cereal, rice, and pasta group **6–11 servings**

*Source:* U.S. Department of Agriculture

Foods are divided into five groups with recommended servings for each:

| Food Group | Servings |
| --- | --- |
| Bread, cereal, rice, and pasta | 6 to 11 |
| Vegetables | 3 to 5 |
| Fruits | 2 to 4 |
| Milk, yogurt, and cheese | 2 to 3 |
| Meat, poultry, fish, dry beans, eggs, and nuts | 2 to 3 |
| Fats, oils, and sweets | Use sparingly |

Eat at least the minimum number of servings from each group, says the American Dietetic Association (ADA). Beyond that, the number of additional servings you'll need depends on your age, sex, health, and amount of physical activity.

For active women, the ADA recommends a total daily calorie intake of about 2,200 calories with about nine servings from the bread group, four servings of vegetables, three of fruit, two to three of milk, and two (total of six ounces) from the meat group.

Active men should consume about 2,800 calories with eleven servings from the bread group, five from the vegetable group, four from the fruit group, two to three from the milk group, and three from the meat group (total of nine ounces).

Going vegetarian as a way to be both healthier and a better athlete can rob the body of iron, inducing iron-deficiency anemia. Susan Kleiner, Ph.D., RD, an affiliate professor at the University of Washington, confirms this: "Many female athletes don't get enough iron. Nutritionists talk about food first, but I recommend an iron supplement if they cannot or will not get enough iron in their diets. Iron and zinc are the minerals most likely to be lacking in an athlete's diet."

"The high-fiber, low-calorie nature of most vegetarian foods may pose a problem for athletes," says the American Council on Exercise (ACE). "Very often the volume of vegetarian foods required to meet their energy needs is greater than their stomach's capacity for food. When energy reserves drop too low, the body will convert its own muscle or protein to compensate for the deficiency, leaving little left over for growth."

One way to shore up calorie consumption is to eat several smaller meals throughout the day or eat carbohydrate- and protein-rich snacks.

If one of your reasons for getting into sports is to lose weight, you might want to think twice before skipping breakfast. According to Chris Rosenbloom, Ph.D., R.D., director of the Sports Nutrition Center at Georgia Tech, skipping breakfast actually slows down the rate at which you burn calories. Eating breakfast, on the other hand, gives the process a boost. "Eating an early morning meal results in calories being expended more rapidly than they would be without eating," he said in the *Penn State Sports Medicine Newsletter.* "Skipping breakfast actually lowers the metabolic rate."

Breakfast is especially important for morning exercise because it replenishes liver glycogen and helps maintain a steady blood-sugar level. Because most players try to make up for the nutrients lost skipping breakfast with carbohydrate-high foods, they never actually compensate for the missed nutrients essential for health.

Examine all the facts before considering following special diets that promise to improve your endurance while helping you lose weight. A case in

## WHAT MATTERS, WHAT DOESN'T

### What Matters
• Getting the RDA of calcium (1,000–1,200 milligrams for men and women, depending on age).

• Taking a multivitamin.

• Taking 250–500 milligrams daily of vitamin C to relieve muscle soreness.

### What Doesn't
• Taking amino acid supplements. (One bite of chicken, for example, gives you 500–700 milligrams of amino acids in a form that's cheaper and tastier.)

• Taking vitamin B supplements. (Additional needs for vitamin B are easily and inexpensively obtained through extra servings of food.)

**SMART DEFINITION**

**Amino acids**

According to the American Council on Exercise: "Building blocks that build, repair, and maintain your body tissues. The body makes nonessential amino acids; others come from foods."

point—the Zone diet advocated by Barry Sears, Ph.D., which recommends a diet high in protein and relatively low in carbohydrate, with almost no dairy products. When the *Penn State Sports Medicine Newsletter* asked leading nutritionists to evaluate Sears's program, it found that "the Zone diet may negatively affect athletic performance because it may contain too little carbohydrate and too few calories. It is a plan contrary to what the most respected sports nutritionists advise, a diet that may diminish athletic performance, and a set of recommendations that may create false hope for people who have life-threatening disease."

If you're thinking of shoring up your diet with supplements, the American Council on Exercise warns that these not only may be unnecessary but even dangerous. That's because there are no established guidelines governing these products, which means companies are not required to offer proof to substantiate their claims. Of particular concern is the use of individual amino acids. Although the council points out that about 9 of the approximately 22 that exist in nature must be present in our diet because the body can't manufacture them on its own, there's no evidence that large doses of a single amino acid is beneficial. In fact, imbalanced amino acid diets created in the lab are associated with poor nutritional effects, such as depressed growth, allergies, headaches, and altered neural functioning. Experts recommend getting amino acids through the protein in foods.

On the other hand, the council does say that moderate quantities of antioxidant vitamins E, C, and beta-carotene in addition to fruits, vegetables and beans "may help get rid of harmful oxidants that can damage cells."

As for chromium picolinate, the supplement much touted as a quick fix to get a lean, muscular physique, ACE says that supporting evidence is nonexistent. But if you're sold on the idea of the supplement, the organization says the estimated safe and adequate daily intake is 50 to 200 micrograms.

When you're trying to fit in a leisure sport on top of an already hectic schedule, it's tempting to eat on the run. Especially when some forms of convenience foods and sports bars are packaged as "energy producing" or "protein supplying." Just how calorie efficient are these foods—do they pack enough energy to justify their calories? Which kind is best suited to give you that needed boost to improve your playing stamina?

The main difference between these products is that protein bars deliver protein while energy bars deliver carbohydrates. Protein bars can pack as much as 30 grams of protein or as little as 4 grams; the less protein they have, the higher their carbohydrate content.

The bars are of value as supplements for athletes who are protein deficient, but are of little benefit for those who get sufficient protein from a balanced diet, and there's no data proving the body actually stores unused protein.

Because their high-carbohydrate content provides fuel to work out, energy bars meet with more approval. But energy bars high in sugar can cause erratic changes in blood sugar levels. For best results, choose energy bars in which the sugar grams are 50 percent or less of the bar's total grams of carbohydrate. The bars should also contain minimal amounts of fat.

"For recreational athletes, it's still better to get their energy needs from food, unless they're really

**SMART MOVE**

What about taking supplements? Advertising by manufacturers often makes it seem as if they're essential to athletic performance. Not so, says the American Council on Exercise. "Supplement manufacturers have promoted many types of bizarre ingredients and concoctions," it says in *Fit Facts*. Some of the most widely used products include individual amino acids, antioxidant vitamins, and trace minerals such as chromium picolinate. While all supplements have the potential to do harm, some are more risky than others.

short on time," says Karen Freeman, M.S., RD, a nutrition consultant in La Jolla and a clinical instructor at the University of California, San Diego, School of Medicine's department of family and preventive medicine. "If you're going to eat an energy bar, you'll need to drink at least two glasses of water with it. And that's hard to do if you're on the run."

Just because smoothies have become a staple at health club snack bars doesn't mean they're performance foods. High in calories, vitamins, minerals, and carbohydrates, smoothies can be part of a balanced diet. "But they aren't to be considered performance foods and shouldn't be eaten immediately before or during competition," Clark warns. "After playing, they're okay."

How soon should you eat before playing? A good rule of thumb is to eat one to six hours beforehand, allowing food time to digest. Otherwise, you could feel bloated and uncomfortable. You may even experience a side stitch often caused by eating too close to the time you play. The best remedy is to back off from playing too hard until the pain eases.

What kinds of food are best to sustain a game? Because carbohydrates give you sustained high energy, the best meals are those high in complex carbohydrates (pasta, potatoes, rice, bread), with a medium amount of protein and minimal fat. Because protein slows digestion of carbs, the combination keeps you from getting hungry quickly. It also prevents a yo-yo effect from a sharp rise and drop in glucose levels so you feel more energetic longer. In addition, when carbs are used as energy, they spare proteins for use in building and repairing tissues.

When you've given the game your all, consider

refueling your energy with more carbohydrate-rich foods. If you're not too hungry, it's okay to fill in temporarily with juice and sports drinks that are high in energy-producing carbohydrates. But the sooner you have a good meal high in complex carbohydrates the better.

# Choosing the Right Shoes

Contrary to what you may think about athletic shoes, differences in design are more than a sales tool. Different sports do actually require differences in support and cushioning; buying a shoe made for aerobic dancing just because it's on sale and using it for another sport isn't a good idea. The purpose of athletic shoes is to protect against both repetitive-use injuries and jarring and twisting that can injure feet, ankles, and knees. Rather than being a fashion statement or an unnecessary extravagance, athletic shoes are the foundation upon which to build safe play. Here are some guidelines in selecting specific types of athletic shoes:

## Aerobic Dancing

Because impact from aerobics can reach up to six times the force of gravity, buy aerobic shoes with plenty of cushioning and shock absorption. Other key criteria are a strong arch, heel support, and sufficiently thick upper leather or strap support to give stability and prevent slips. A high toe box will protect against toe and nail irritation. Don't even

**F.Y.I.**

Athletic shoes wear out more quickly than you may think. To prevent injuries from worn-out shoes, the *Penn State Sports Medicine Newsletter* suggests:

• Replacing running shoes every 350 to 500 miles

• Replacing walking shoes every 1,000 miles

• Replacing aerobic shoes after six months

During the first month of wearing new shoes, fully unlace and then retighten the strings weekly to maintain support.

think about doing double duty with running shoes, the most popular kind of athletic shoe in America. Not only do these have an acute outside flare that could put you at greater risk of injury in sports requiring side-by-side motion, but they also lift the heel too high for aerobics.

## Racquet Sports

Make sure shoes are designed for racquet sports, have extra rubber on the tops of the toes to prevent wear, and have good support so you can perform quick maneuvers without damaging your knees.

## Golf

Shoes should have comfortable cushioning and arch support for walking plus advanced technological innovations such as graphite shank reinforcements to keep them light but strong.

## Cycling

Use cross-training shoes with support across the arch and instep, as well as heel lift. Combination cycling-hiking shoes are also recommended.

## Skiing and Ice Skating

Your footware should have a comfortable, snug fit to prevent injury from the pressure exerted by the constant forward motion and sideways movement of skating and the quick turns of skiing. Hand-me downs that are too tight can cause blisters and abrasions while inhibiting circulation in the lower extremities so that feet get cold. Loose boots and skates can irritate toes, and leave the ankle vulnerable to sprains, strains, or fractures. Cross-country skiing requires footwear more like a bicycle shoe than a downhill boot and must be properly fitted to avoid irritating the balls of the feet.

## Walking

Look for good heel support and flexibility at the ball of the foot to provide traction and propel you forward safely. Shoes for fitness walking should have additional cushioning.

# Shoe Shopping

If you've always thought all sports shoes are created equal and that all shoes are equally adaptable to all sports, you're likely to get your playing career off on the wrong foot. Here's some advice from the American Podiatric Medical Society.

• Because most athletic shoes are manufactured abroad where sizing parameters vary significantly even within the same single factory, buy shoes based on how they fit rather than how they're sized.

• For best fit, shop in the afternoon so shoes will accommodate normal swelling that occurs during the day. Feet can swell as much as 5 percent during the day.

• Always have your foot size measured wearing the sport-specific sock you'll be wearing.

• If you have foot problems, pick a shoe in which the back (called the counter) is rigid.

**F.Y.I.**

Different types of feet need different types of shoes. Here are some guidelines from the American Council on Exercise:

• Choose shoes according to foot type. People with high-arched feet have different needs in terms of shoe support than those with flat feet.

• If you have high-arched feet, choose shoes with greater shock absorption.

• Flat feet require shoes with less cushioning but greater support and heel control.

• Shoes should be as wide as possible across the forefoot without allowing slippage in the heel.

• Athletic shoes no longer require a breaking-in period. However, they should be replaced after three to six months of regular use because cushioning wears out.

• If you wear orthotics, try shoes on with them.

• Don't wear athletic shoes for sports other than the ones for which they're designed. Different sports have different shoe needs.

Carol Frey, M.D., an orthopedic surgeon at the University of Southern California, and Utah Jazz pro basketball team podiatrist Dr. Michael Low offer these tips on fit and shoe type when buying new or used athletic shoes:

• The shoe's heel cup should fit snugly; the rest of the shoe should not.

• Athletic shoes don't require a breaking in period and won't stretch out, so they must fit well when you first buy them.

• Feet with high arches require thicker soles and padding in running and court shoes.

• Feet with low arches (flat feet) require thinner, stiffer soles in running and court shoes.

# Socks

Depending on their construction, socks can actually dissipate some of the damaging forces to which your feet are exposed in play. According to the American Academy of Podiatric Sports Medicine (AAPSM), the best socks are made of synthetic fibers like acrylic. They keep feet cool and maintain their shape without stretching. Acrylics also minimize formation of friction blisters, the most common foot injury plaguing athletes. To further protect against blisters, be sure that socks fit well without crimping or folding.

When it's important to keep your feet warm, with sports like skating and skiing, a sock made of a wool-synthetic blend provides superior insulation. A new synthetic called Thermax is also recommended.

Of course, shoes aren't the only equipment that needs careful selection to keep you safe. Racquets that are too large for your hand, and golf clubs or skis that are the wrong length are typical of equipment mistakes that can set you up for injury.

# Getting Started with Lessons and Clubs

Of course, how extensively you condition depends on how much time you have. "To minimize risk for overuse injury if you're determined to start playing next week, do some general overall conditioning," says Lee Rice. "If the sport is unfamiliar, lessons are an excellent way to shorten the learning curve. They'll also decrease your chance of developing biomechanical faults that will result in injury by overstressing certain areas of your body."

Working with a pro, coach, or trainer will give you pointers on what to avoid in posture, body balance, and alignment, especially if you're untrained and not well-conditioned. If, for example, you're beginning a sport like softball, a trainer watching you throw can analyze your form and recommend changes to help prevent your developing bad habits and suffering injury. By observing you on a treadmill, a pro can pick up asymmetries in motion that will make you vulnerable to becoming hurt in sports like running, squash, and tennis that stress the legs and lower body.

Sometimes the best help for an athletic injury doesn't come from a physician. Treating recurrent bouts of tennis elbow with anti-inflammatory medications is only a Band-Aid approach. If you continue to injure your elbow because of poor backhand form, what you really need is coaching.

A wide variety of facilities offer group instructions to get you started at very reasonable prices. To locate such organizations in your community, check the monthly listings at the *Learning Annex,* YMCAs and YWCAs, JCCs, Department of Parks and Recreation, extension courses at local colleges and universities, adult schools, and private tennis and golf clubs.

## THE BOTTOM LINE

Before starting to play sports or beginning a new one, get a fix on your own limitations with an appraisal of your health and baseline fitness. Develop a smart conditioning program to improve duration, frequency, and intensity of play. Put special emphasis on stretching and toning the parts of your body most under stress in a specific sport. Learn to have a positive mental attitude that forgives errors and allows you to learn a new sport at a safe pace. Pay attention to your equipment; buying the right shoes enhances enjoyment of leisure sports by minimizing exposure to injury.

# CHAPTER 2

# Pain: What It Means and How to Treat It

**THE KEYS**

• Misconceptions about pain can lead to more serious injuries such as the overuse syndrome.

• Learning to administer basic first aid for sports injuries will keep you and other players safe.

• Returning to the game before an injury is completely healed can cause a domino effect of more complicated injuries.

• Learning how to distinguish between minor and major injuries and when it's safe to resume playing can prevent injuries from escalating in seriousness.

• Avoid dehydration by drinking eight glasses of fluids a day, preferably water. Compensate for caffeinated beverages by alternating each with a decaf.

• If an injury sidelines you, harness the healing power of your mind for a quicker rebound.

Every new activity—including beginning a new leisure sport—has a host of new skills associated with its mastery. To perfect your technique, you must learn what constitutes good form and what mistakes to avoid. Since mistakes in form can lead to accidents and injuries, you must also learn how to recognize the difference between minor and more serious injuries, how to treat them, and the ins and outs of developing secondary injuries. Occasionally, athletes find an injury is more extensive than initially thought, and find themselves dealing with the physical and psychological ramifications of recuperation.

# Myths and Facts about Pain

Often it's not what we know but what we think we know that gets us into trouble. That's particularly the case in deciphering the messages our body gives us about pain. Misinterpret or ignore the symptoms and an innocuous incident can quickly escalate into something serious. Here's a rundown of the common misconceptions and the facts behind them.

**Myth:** No pain, no gain.
**Fact:** "If your conditioning and training programs and the way in which you perform a sport are correct, you shouldn't ordinarily experience pain," says Denise Wiksten, Ph.D., A.T.C., assistant professor of exercise and nutrition at San Diego State University. "Pain is our body's way of telling us

something is wrong," she warns. "It's a protective mechanism telling us to stop what we're doing to see what's gone wrong."

**Myth:** Pain and soreness are the same.
**Fact:** "Pain and soreness are distinctly different," says Wiksten. "Feeling sore after conditioning exercises like weight training indicates that you've worked your muscles in a healthy way. But if soreness is so painful that it interferes with performing your daily routine, you've overworked. Take at least a day off to rest and recuperate those muscles."

**Myth:** Always work through pain.
**Fact:** "Pain is an impetus to stop playing and ask questions," says Wiksten. "What's causing the pain? Are you wearing incorrect shoes for the sport? Is your form off? Have you skipped your warm-up so that you're straining or tearing muscle tissue?"

# Self-Diagnosing Pain

Just as important as sorting out misconceptions about pain is the ability to distinguish between those injuries that will disappear quickly on their own, those that need first aid, and those that require additional attention from a physician.

If you or someone you're playing with is hurt, the first rule of thumb is to give yourself enough time to assess an injury before toughing it out or going on with the game. If you've fallen, don't move until you feel you can do so without collapsing. Don't let being injured embarrass you into moving prematurely.

A National Federation of Professional Trainers'

**SMART MOVE**

"The first warning signal an athlete gets indicating something is wrong is pain," says Thomas Wickiewicz, M.D., an orthopedic surgeon and chief of the sports medicine department at the Hospital for Special Surgery in New York City. "He must then decide whether the pain is just soreness from exercise or whether it's a sharp sensation coming from a joint. If the joint hurts while playing or becomes worse, he should have an evaluation by a physician. The second symptom to pay attention to is swelling. Is he experiencing just puffiness that disappears quickly or is the swelling occurring in a joint? If it's the latter, the injury could be serious and must be examined by a health professional."

article, "Minor Injury Treatment," indicated that injuries to muscles and ligaments have four characteristics—pain, warmth, redness, and swelling. The symptoms are more intense in more serious injuries. "For example, a minor injury involving the tearing of a few muscle fibers will have slight pain; the skin over the muscle will be slightly warm; little or no noticeable redness and generally no swelling. On the other hand, all four characteristics will be very pronounced in a very severe muscle strain."

# Injury Checklist

To appraise whether or not pain will resolve on its own in a few days or whether you need immediate medical attention, the Rose Medical Center in Denver, Colorado and the Columbia/HCA Healthcare Corporation's Sports Medicine Page advise asking yourself these questions:

- Is the pain mild, moderate, or severe?

- Is it becoming worse?

- Does it increase with slight motion?

- Has a bone protruded from the skin?

- Is swelling worsening quickly?

- Is the area black and blue?

- Can I walk or move the injured part?

- Does it feel numb?

• Is the area below the injury cold, numb, or white in color?

• Does the injury feel better with rest?

If you have minimal pain and can move without more or serious pain, and there is minimal swelling, your injuries should respond to basic first aid.

# When to Call the Doctor

If you've answered yes to some or most of these questions, get medical help immediately. When pain actually increases with every little movement or you're unable to walk, or the pain is really severe, generally the injury is serious.

If you heard a "pop" or "snap" when the accident occurred, you probably hurt a bone, ligament, tendon, or a combination of these. And if you can't move the injured body part, you've probably either broken a bone, dislocated a joint, or suffered a serious joint or muscle strain. Numbness, on the other hand, may indicate an injury to a nerve. Change in color, a noticeable deformity, or an increase in swelling also indicates a more severe condition that merits intervention by a physician.

Regardless of whether your initial assessment indicates the damage is minimal, or if you're waiting for medical attention to treat a more extensive injury, applying basic first aid can prevent problems from escalating.

## SMART MOVE

Earl Grubbs, M.D., a physician at Columbia Eastside Medical Center in Atlanta, offers these precautions for all emergency situations: "Don't delay in getting to the emergency room. Don't go home and soak in a hot tub, which can lead to further swelling and bleeding. Don't eat before going to the hospital because eating will delay the surgery for six hours."

# Step 1: The RICE Formula

According to the *Healthwise Handbook,* injuries to muscles, ligaments, tendons, or bones are treated through a two-part process. The first step is to quickly control swelling and relieve pain by applying RICE (rest, ice, compression, elevation).

• **Rest:** If you've injured any part of your leg, stay off your feet for 24 to 48 hours. Immobilize any part of your hand, arm, or shoulder that may be sprained with a sling.

• **Ice:** To reduce pain, swelling, and slow bleeding into the injured tissues, apply ice hourly for 10 minutes for the first 72 hours if possible or at least 15 to 20 minutes three times a day. Protect your skin from being burned by putting the ice pack on top of a damp cloth.

• **Compression:** Increase the pressure inside the injured tissue to slow down bleeding and swelling with an elastic bandage. Wrap the bandage firmly, being careful not to cut off circulation. Warning: Even if the bandage relieves so much of the discomfort that you feel able to return to your normal activities, don't. Give the injury time to rest and recuperate; a day or two is recommended.

• **Elevation:** Keep the affected joint above the level of your heart by propping it up with pillows when sitting or lying down.

When a foot or ankle is injured, some athletes and trainers actually prefer to immerse the injury in ice for 20 minutes rather than apply an ice pack. Though this cold therapy (cryotherapy) reduces pain, some are concerned that its use actually hampers agility, making it dangerous for athletes to exercise afterward.

Not to worry says a joint study by the Department of Orthopedic Surgery at Washington University, Barnes West County Hospital in St. Louis, Indiana State University, and the Krannert School of Physical Therapy at the University of Indianapolis. Although athletes' performance was slightly slower after the immersion, the study found that cryotherapy both for joints and muscles is safe and effective.

However, one of the authors did recommend that "due to altered sensation and subsequent apprehension, vigorous exercise and athletic competition following cold therapy should not begin until athletes feel they are ready."

## Splints

An injury that looks suspiciously like a broken or fractured bone should be splinted immediately, a procedure that's relatively simple. To immobilize the limb so that it can't bend, use a belt or rope to tie it to a stiff support like rolled up newspapers. Alternately, some injuries like a broken toe or finger can be taped to the next toe. Always splint from a joint above the fracture to the joint below. For example, splint a broken knee from above the knee to below the ankle.

# Step 2: The MSA Formula

After the initial pain and swelling have subsided (and you've clearance from a physician if you required medical attention), the *Healthwise Handbook*

**SMART MOVE**

Bryant Stamford, Ph.D., writes in *The Physician and Sports Medicine* that cold therapy may not be advised for people who are

• Highly cold sensitive and incapable of tolerating prolonged periods of icing.

• Highly tolerant to cold or prefer to "tough out" injuries. They may injure themselves by applying ice too long.

• Suffering from diabetes, Raynaud's phenomenon, or other problems in the blood vessels near the skin that can diminish blood flow.

**SMART DEFINITION**

**Muscle cramps**

A painful muscle contraction or stiffness that either lasts too long or won't loosen up. It is sometimes called a charley horse when it is in the upper leg.

recommends beginning rehabilitation with MSA (movement, strength, alternate activity).

• **Movement:** To restore full range of motion, try exercising the joint lightly with mild stretches one to two days after the injury. This will also help to prevent scar tissue formation.

• **Strength:** After swelling has disappeared and you can move the joint fully, slowly add strengthening exercises. (Consult your physician, coach, or a trainer at your local gym for specific advice.)

• **Alternate Activities:** During this process maintain your overall fitness by adding cross-training sports that don't strain the injury. Try swimming if you're recovering from sore feet, or take up cycling if you have injured elbows. Take your time returning to the sport in which you became injured.

## Muscle Cramps

Some injuries may be nothing more than muscle cramps. Though they may be so painful they stop you cold when you're exercising, cramps in themselves are not serious. The result of becoming oxygen-depleted, cramps may be caused by a build-up of lactic acid that can cause difficulty in moving. Muscle cramps may also be triggered by:

• Over- or underuse of muscles

• Insufficient warm-up prior to play

• Dehydration

• Insufficient potassium and magnesium in diet

Cramps are particularly common among swimmers, but can be remedied by stretching. Whenever you experience a charley horse, stop whatever you're doing and ease the pain in your aching muscle with a slow stretch. If, for example, your calf cramps up, a common occurrence in sports, straighten your leg and point your foot and toes up for a good thorough stretch.

# Your First-Aid Kit

To be able to apply basic first aid, you need both know-how and the means to execute it. Since no one can predict where and when an injury may occur, it makes smart sports sense to have a portable first-aid kit close at hand, if at all possible. Here's what to include:

- Ace bandages

- Butterfly bandages

- Band-Aids

- Gauze

- Over-the-counter pain medications like Tylenol, Motrin, or aspirin

- Peroxide or Betadine for wound cleansing

- Antibiotic ointment

- Chemical cold bags

The good news is that you may never need to use this kit if you prepare for play intelligently. That means incorporating into your sporting activity a proper warm-up and cool down; a good conditioning program to build strength, flexibility, and endurance; and help from coaches or trainers as to proper technique and form, and the right equipment.

# Pain Remedies

A variety of over-the-counter (OTC) analgesics can relieve pain associated with athletic injuries. Which ones you choose depend on your stomach's tolerance and whether or not you also need anti-inflammatory relief.

For those suffering both pain and inflammation, aspirin is a good choice. To prevent against stomach irritation, use buffered or enteric aspirin. However, its use is counterindicated if you're already taking other anti-inflammatory medications like ibuprofen.

Ibuprofen, a nonsteroidal anti-inflammatory (NSAID) is the active ingredient in medications like Advil and is effective in relieving pain and inflammation. Tylenol holds the patent for the ingredient acetaminophen, which relieves pain without reducing swelling.

Be cautious about using prescription muscle relaxants, which can make you drowsy.

To relieve exercise-related muscle soreness and decrease recovery time between workouts, you may want to try l-carnitine supplements. According to a 1996 study reported in the *International Journal of Sports Medicine,* the supplement ups oxygen delivery to muscles while speeding up the elimination of waste products accumulated during exercise. Results were based on three weeks of daily doses of three grams.

New research from Yale University and the National Cancer Institute suggests that a topical cream made from capsaicin, a substance found in red peppers, may actually diminish the number of pain signals sent to the brain. Capsaicin creams stimulate nerve cells to overproduce a chemical substance that transmits pain signals. Used several times daily, these creams appear to deplete the nerve cells' supply, thus decreasing the amount of pain messages and diminishing pain. In some people, this also results in increased ability to move painful joints.

One of the minor side effects of these creams is a burning sensation to the area where the cream is applied.

# Myths and Facts about Treating Injuries

Old wives' tales heard growing up often prevent us from getting the right help in the right way at the right time. This misinformation can delay injury rehabilitation and even make injuries worse. Here's what to look out for:

**Myth:** Something is broken only if it can't be moved.
**Fact:** That's a myth that often keeps people from having fractures treated when they are fresh.

**SMART DEFINITION**

The *Healthwise Handbook* offers these useful definitions:

**Strain**

An injury caused by overstretching a muscle.

**Sprain**

An injury to the muscle and the ligaments, tendons, or soft tissues around a joint.

**Fracture**

A break in a bone.

Among the types of fractures with which you can still walk are small chip fractures of foot or ankle-bones, and toe fractures.

**Myth:** A broken toe doesn't need immediate attention.
**Fact:** Like fractures of other bones, toes need immediate attention. "Many people develop post-fracture deformity of a toe, which in turn results in formation of a painfully deformed toe with a most painful corn," warns the American Podiatric Medical Association. "If not properly treated, displaced breaks won't heal right."

**Myth:** Soak foot or ankle injures in hot water immediately.
**Fact:** "Never use heat or hot water if a fracture, sprain or dislocation is suspected," warns the APMA. "Because heat promotes increased blood flow, it triggers greater swelling which in turn places greater pressure on the nerves and additional pain." Always apply ice first.

**Myth:** All a severely sprained ankle requires to heal is an elastic bandage.
**Fact:** "Ankle sprains often indicate torn or severely overstretched ligaments, which may require X-ray, casts, splints and/or physical therapy," says the APMA. Occasionally, surgery may be indicated.

# Preventing Injuries

In an ideal world, athletes would preclude the possibility of becoming injured by following some commonsense guidelines to minimize the possibility of their occurrence: Here is a rundown of smart ways to keep yourself fit and able to play:

• Alternate hard play with easy play to let your body recuperate. For example, if you play tennis, alternate a more demanding game of singles with easy-going rallies or a less intense competition of doubles.

• Relax muscles under stress by cross training. If, for example, your primary sport is swimming, rest your upper body muscles on alternate days by jogging or biking.

• Take action immediately if you experience pain. Cut back on play and use ice and other home remedies to keep a twinge from developing into more extensive problems.

• Warm up for five minutes between games.

• Women are at higher risk for knee injuries and should protect their knees by developing strong thigh muscles with conditioning exercises for the legs.

# Emergency Care Errors

Sometimes misinformation coupled with the urgency of an injury leads to mistakes in emergency care that can be serious. The *Penn State Sports Medicine Newsletter* has identified four such errors that can exacerbate injury.

## Head Injuries

If a concussion hasn't been ruled out, further injury can be caused by allowing an athlete to get back into play right after a head injury occurs or moving her too soon.

## Bleeding

If a tourniquet has been applied too tightly to stop bleeding, it could cut circulation dangerously. On the other hand, failure to apply sufficient pressure won't contain the bleeding. A good rule of thumb is to go to an emergency room immediately if a bandage becomes saturated with blood.

## Sprains/Strains

Unless an athlete suffers a muscle spasm, walking off an injury instead of resting can make an injury worse.

## Dislocations

Rather than try to relocate dislocations, immobilize the injury with a splint. Anesthetize the pain with an ice pack, and get to a physician immediately. "We don't even relocate a dislocation at the hospital until we take an X-ray to rule out a fracture," said Earl Grubbs, an emergency room physician in Atlanta.

Delays in getting to the emergency room when a physician's attention is critical can also result in making an injury more severe. If you must transport an injured, bleeding individual, don't remove any dressing that's been applied to the wound, regardless of the bandages' condition. What you want to avoid is reopening the wound. Don't remove any large objects imbedded in the wound to avoid triggering blood loss from a critical blood vessel or artery.

# Secondary Injuries

The effect of an injury may outlast the pain it initially caused. Just because symptoms seem to have disappeared doesn't necessarily mean you're ready to return to playing at your previous intensity.

Researches studying the domino effect of injuries are discovering that primary damage to a joint or muscle may cause secondary weakness or alteration in body mechanics that affect athletic performance. At the University of Buffalo, Harold Burton, Ph.D., an associate professor in the department of physical therapy, exercise, and nutrition services, is concerned that untreated injuries, those that are incompletely healed or which have affected changes in gait can predispose athletes to additional problems.

"For example, if a runner injures the quadriceps, there is a possibility that he will alter his running mechanics for periods up to four days after the injuries," he says.

According to Burton, because the "chain of events required to execute sports skills consists of head-to-toe links," researchers are concerned that injuries may have longer-lasting implications affecting other muscle groups. To compensate for primary injury, the athlete may misuse or overuse other muscle groups. To prevent this domino effect of more subtle and potentially more debilitating injuries, remember this three-fold approach to dealing with accidents:

## SMART MOVE

"The most important part of treating an injury is to address the cause, not just the symptom of pain," says Denise Wiksten, Ph.D., A.T.C., assistant professor of exercise and nutrition at San Diego State University. "Is the pain due to wrong shoes, poor posture, and incorrect gait?

"I put them through the drill. We look at the surfaces they're running; examine their body mechanics; and dissect their training habits. Sometimes it is as simple as running on a 'crowned' surface—a road that's raised in the middle and flanked by a gully on each side. One foot goes further down into the gully, causing problems in that knee. Examining the cause and remedying the underlying problems, rather than just fixing the symptoms, is the sensible way to treat an injury."

Joe Nichols, a 19-year-old student at San Diego State University, liked to socialize in the evening over a few beers with friends. But the next day, by the time he'd hit the tennis courts to work out with the team, he'd chased away the beers with several cups of strong java. As the afternoon heated up, Joe became increasingly nauseous and started to perspire heavily.

Joe said: "I never realized that the alcohol and coffee I drank in the last 24 hours could actually cause dehydration. I took a break in the shade and tried drinking a glass of water. When it was clear that I could keep it down, I drank another two glasses. By then, the sweating had stopped and I felt back to normal. From now on, I'm going to be a lot more careful about what I drink before I play sports!"

**1.** Seek advice or treatment for an injury as soon as it happens.

**2.** To minimize the chances of suffering other indirect injuries, reduce the intensity and duration of exercise even if you're able to continue playing.

**3.** Once recovered, be sure you haven't developed a compensatory change in your gait or form that could signal future problems.

# Preventing Dehydration

Most Americans get about three-quarters of the fluid they need. The problem becomes more acute for athletes because playing sports requires even greater hydration.

One of the villains is caffeine. Found in coffee, tea, and soft drinks, caffeine is a diuretic that causes loss of fluid through increased urination. Eight glasses of fluid a day—part of which comes from coffee, tea, soft drinks, or alcohol—actually equates to just three glasses of usable fluid. The rest is excreted as urine. The added demands for fluid during sports makes the problem more acute.

Susan Kleiner, author of *Power Eating,* advises, "Most caffeine users don't drink their beverage of choice just once a day. My recommendation is that every eight-ounce caffeinated drink should be replaced with an eight-ounce cup of fluid that does not contain caffeine."

Kleiner also points out that caffeine content varies in amount from drink to drink, and that some high-octane alternative beverages like Jolt and Surge contain substantially more. If you're going to count on these to produce energy highs, be sure to drink even more noncaffeinated beverages to mitigate their effect on water loss.

According to the American Dietetic Association's *Complete Food and Nutrition Guide,* a 150-pound athlete can lose the equivalent of six eight-ounce glasses of water in just one hour as a result of sweating during exercise. To prevent dehydration when you're exercising, drink lots of fluids even if you don't feel thirsty.

"Dehydration can be cumulative," Freeman warns. "If you're not drinking enough fluids, you may not feel the affect for the first one or two days. But by the third or fourth days, you'll begin to exhibit fatigue, one of the signs of dehydration."

## Dehydration Warnings

What are the signs that an athlete's becoming dehydrated? Here are some warning signs from the American College of Sports Medicine's booklet *Stay Cool to Perform Best*:

**Acute Signs (can occur within one hour)**

- Nausea
- Poor concentration
- Flushed skin
- Light-headedness

**Chronic Signs***

- Loss of appetite
- Dark yellow urine
- Little or no urination
- Muscle cramps

* If you experience these symptoms, take fluids, cool down in the shade, and if necessary, consult a coach or a physician.

A new study in the *Journal of Science and Medicine in Sports* reports that fluid replacement guidelines may need to be adjusted to accommodate the differences in gender. The study examined male and female runners and found that fluid loss and replacement needs among the men were two times as great as among the women.

"It's important for each athlete to assess his or her own fluid loss based on weight before and after strenuous exercise," advises Mindy Millard-Stafford, associate professor in the department of health and performance sciences at Georgia Tech in the *Georgia Tech Sports Medicine & Performance Newsletter.* Individual differences can also be affected by how well trained an athlete is, environmental conditions, and the effects of the menstrual cycle on hydration, she points out.

What types of fluids best keep you hydrated? Water, fruit juices, and sports drinks all do the trick. If you play continuously for less than an hour, the ADA recommends water, sports drinks, or juices. Before playing, drink two eight-ounce glasses of fluid, but stay away from soft drinks high in sugar because they can cause blood sugar and energy to plummet just when you need them the most.

"To be sure you're actually getting the fluids you need, check the color of your urine," says Freeman. "If you're properly hydrated, urine should be pale yellow to clear. A dark yellow color is a definite sign of dehydration. However, vitamin supplements (if you're taking them) can change the color of urine so it's harder to tell if you're getting enough fluids."

To lower your body temperature when exercising, drink fluids that have been cooled. Contrary to myth, a cool temperature won't cause muscle cramps, says the ADA. Lack of fluids will.

Sport drinks can play an important role in keeping your fluid intake up, but not all sports drinks are equally nutritious. "In selecting a sports drink, it's important to determine sugar content," says Freeman. "Choose those that have no more than 50 to 70 calories per 8 ounces."

After exercising, you may want to stay away from carbonated beverages. According to a study by the Gatorade Sports Science Institute, carbonated beverages shouldn't be used to replace fluid lost during exercise because they have a lower "drink acceptability" level. Among other things, they make you feel your thirst is quenched faster, causing you to drink less fluid than actually needed to hydrate your body after playing.

# Illnesses from Playing in Hot Weather

Performing sports in hot weather and exerting yourself in summerlike conditions can cause three very different types of illnesses—heat cramps, heat exhaustion, and heat stroke. All three, however, can result in serious injuries and health complications, so a little knowledge and a few precautions will go a long way toward keeping you healthy and active in the hot months.

## Muscle Cramps

Even if you've drunk plenty of water, you can still experience heat cramps if your electrolyte balance is low. This typically occurs in athletes who fail to

**STREET SMARTS**

"My goal in doing sports was to lose weight," says Nan G., a 26-year-old R.N. "Even though I knew it was important to be hydrated, I never liked to drink fluids before playing because it made me feel bloated. When I consulted a nutritionist about my weight-loss goals, she persuaded me to substitute Gatorade for food prior to playing. She said it would give me more energy by providing a glucose boost. I was petrified that the calories would actually cause me to gain weight. Finally, I agreed to try drinking 4 ounces every 15 minutes during the hour I did aerobic dancing. Not only did it give me more energy, but it actually reduced the hunger I normally felt after exercise. It just goes to show that a little bit of calories can go a long way!"

## Time to Fuel Up!

How much and what kinds of fluids do the trick? If you're involved in rigorous activity, the American College of Sports Medicine and the American Dietetic Association's *Complete Food & Nutrition Guide* recommend fluids on the following schedule:

| When | How Much |
|---|---|
| 2 to 2½ hours before activity | At least 2 cups of nonalcoholic fluids (water, juice, milk, or some other fluid) |
| Just prior to or up to 15 minutes before | 2 cups of water or sports drink |
| Every 15 minutes during activity | 5 to 10 ounces of fluid |
| After activity | 2 cups of water or, preferably, a high-carbohydrate drink such as fruit juice for every pound lost during your activity; continue to drink fluids throughout the day until you return to your pre-exercise weight |

add dried fruits, fruit juices, or electrolyte solutions to their diet when playing in high heat and humidity. "They'll come in with fairly dramatic muscle cramps. Often these are in the abdomen, although the entire body can be affected," reports Knox Todd, M.D., in the Emory University School of Medicine's Division of Emergency Medicine in the *Columbia Sports Medicine News*.

Heat cramps usually respond to cooling and intravenous saline solutions.

## Heat Exhaustion

More severe is heat exhaustion experienced by players unaccustomed to high heat and humidity. Though the symptoms of nausea, vomiting, headache and pronounced fatigue can be frightening, most people recover quickly when they get out of the heat and start replacing fluids and lost electrolytes with dried fruit, fruit juices, sports drinks, and electrolyte solutions.

## Heat Stroke

When body temperature gets so extremely high that sweating in itself can't cool the body down, heat stroke develops. An extremely dangerous condition, often accompanied by symptoms of confusion and neurological impairment, heat stroke requires emergency care to reduce body temperature. Sometimes hospitalization is also necessary.

If you're going to be playing in high heat and humidity, give your body about 10 days of preparation to acclimatize. Gradually expose your body to heat stress by playing under hot conditions.

# Bouncing Back Physically

Little is more dispiriting than having to take time off from your favorite sport for an extended period of time. Even though you can't play, there are steps you can take to improve your game.

**F.Y.I.**

The American College of Sports Medicine offers these tips to keep you healthy playing sports in hot weather:

• Pouring water over your head won't help replenish the body's fluids.

• Drinks that are "lightly flavored and sweetened and contain sodium" will encourage athletes to drink more.

• Keep your sweat-soaked shirt on even during breaks because it cools the body better than a dry shirt.

• Play sports in the morning or in the evening when the temperature drops.

• Break down the elements in playing a sport into specific skill patterns. "These can be practiced by using sport-specific drills," says Michael J. Mullin, A.T.C, P.T.A., at the Stone Clinic. Once you analyze the sport, itemizing the different components involved in playing, get your physician's okay to practice those aspects while you recuperate.

• Exercise other muscle groups used in your favorite sport while the injured ones are recuperating. Suppose, for example, a golfer injured an ankle or knee and is told to keep weight off the affected joints. "That's an opportunity to work on back strengthening with exercises focused on good posture, rotation, and flexibility," says Mullin.

• Keep your mind on the game by visualizing techniques to sharpen your performance. For instance, visualize the perfect backhand swing in tennis to return a ball forcefully over the net.

• Once it's safe to begin using the body parts you've injured, your physician or physical therapist will recommend sport-specific exercises designed to rehabilitate your injury so you can play again. Take it slow and don't overdo; otherwise you run the risk of an overuse injury, undoing all your efforts at rehab.

# Bouncing Back Psychologically

One of the toughest parts of becoming injured is coping with the psychological fallout from being sidelined. When you've put considerable effort into learning a leisure sport, time out of the game to rehab an injury is a significant loss. In their book *Rehabilitation in Sports Medicine,* sports psychologists Dave Yukelson, Ph.D., and John Heil, Ph.D., say the adjustment is not unlike some of the stages associated with death and dying described by Elizabeth Kubler-Ross. Particularly when it comes to the cycle of distress, denial, and determined coping, a process that can falter with each rehab setback.

Here is where learning to turn negative, self-defeating thoughts into positive self-talk can be very effective. For example, rather than focusing on things that are out of your control (like watching others improve while you can't train), you should "focus on short-term rehabilitation goals that affirm the progress you're making," say the authors. "Learning to spot negative interior dialogue is the first step in gaining control of self-defeating attitudes."

To move successfully from injury through rehab and back into the game, it's essential to apply the same skills used in play—setting goals and developing plans to deal with potential setbacks.

Here are some suggestions:

• Think of your injury and pain as things that will go away.

• Write down some positive statements about your ability to cope and recover.

• Repeat these affirmations daily.

• Use your desire to recover to help you connect with your own healing power.

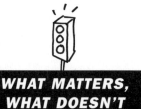

## WHAT MATTERS, WHAT DOESN'T

### What Matters

• Taking the time to assess an injury before deciding to remain in the game.

• Applying basic first aid while waiting for emergency care.

• Gauging the seriousness of an injury by looking for changes in skin color, swelling, or sensitivity to movement.

### What Doesn't

• Being embarrassed because you think you've "let the side down" by stopping to care for an injury.

• Worrying that immersing a hurt foot or ankle in ice will interfere with agility upon returning to the game. It doesn't.

**SMART SOURCES**

The following organizations can help you find out more about their specialties and help you locate one of their members in your area:

The American Academy
   of Orthopaedic
   Surgeons
6300 N. River Road
Rosemont, IL. 60018-
   4262
(800) 346-AAOS
www.aaos.org

The American
   Orthopaedic Foot
   and Ankle Society
1216 Pine Street
Suite 201
Seattle, WA 98101
(206) 223-1120
www.aofas.org

The American Chiro-
   practic Association
1701 Clarendon Blvd.
Arlington, VA 22209-
   2700
(703) 327-8800
www.amerchiro.org

American Physical
   Therapy Association
www.apata.edoc.com

• Try to maintain your sense of identity and importance by doing things that help you feel good about yourself.

# How to Choose a Sports Medicine Practitioner

Sports injuries are treated by a variety of physicians. Though there is no separate board certification in sports medicine, physicians already board-certified in pediatrics, emergency medicine, family practice, and internal medicine are eligible to qualify for a certificate in sports medicine by passing a special exam. The simplest way to ascertain whether or not a physician has qualified for this additional certification is to ask his/her office before making an appointment. Often a particular specialist will refer you to a different specialist more appropriate for treating your condition.

Depending on the type of injury you have, you may also want to consider consulting one of the following:

• **Orthopedic surgeons** are trained to treat disorders of the bones and joints, and the muscles, tendons, and ligaments associated with them, both with and without surgery.

• **Osteopaths** are fully licensed physicians who specialize in structural diagnosis and spinal manipulation therapy.

• **Physiatrists** specialize in the diagnosis, prevention, and treatment of musculoskeletal disorders.

• **Podiatrists** are Doctors of Podiatric Medicine specializing in diagnosing, treating, and preventing diseases and malfunctions of the foot.

• **Physical therapists** are not physicians; however, they are trained and licensed to use most of the same techniques employed by physiatrists. They cannot diagnosis disease or prescribe drugs.

# Should You Choose an Alternative Medicine Practitioner?

Because more Americans are seeking out alternative medicine practitioners than ever before, some insurance plans have actually begun covering some of the costs associated with their patients' alternative health care. The effectiveness of various treatment therapies like acupuncture in reducing pain have also come under scrutiny by such prestigious organizations as the National Institutes of Health (NIH). In 1997, the agency issued a report concluding that acupuncture "merits inclusion in the comprehensive treatment for twelve conditions, including tennis elbow, low back pain, asthma, and carpal tunnel syndrome."

In their 1994 report establishing uniform treatment guidelines for low back pain, the Agency for Health Care Policy and Research (AHCPR) recommended chiropractic manipulation for the short-

**SMART SOURCES**

The North American Society of Acupuncture and Alternative Medicine
816 Frederick Road
Catonsville, MD 21228
www.nasa-altmed.com

## THE BOTTOM LINE

Learning how to read the severity of injuries and when it's safe to resume play can prevent injuries from escalating in seriousness. While it's tempting to continue playing through pain when winning, failing to monitor and respond to an injury will only make it worse, lengthening healing time. Athletes who push themselves to the point of pain because they've bought into the "no pain, no gain" myth are sabotaging both their performance and overall well-being.

Equally important is learning how to prevent injuries by alternating how you play and train and by regular warm-ups and stretching.

Knowing how to treat injuries and the dos and don'ts of transporting the injured is as vital as learning CPR.

If you are injured, harness the healing power of your mind for a quicker rebound.

term relief of low back pain. In fact, they found that manipulation appears superior to conventional care.

With these findings in mind, you may want to consider incorporating alternative practitioners such as those practicing acupuncture, Oriental medicine, chiropractic care, and other modalities into your program.

# Treating Common Injuries: Skin, Head, and Back

Because most recreational sports are non-contact events, most weekend athletes seldom give a second thought to the possibility of ever becoming injured. They forget that playing outdoors can result in a burn, or that playing team sports or using a racquet to hit a ball has the potential of delivering a blow to the eyes or any other part of the body. They forget about the fact that they've spent most of their time sitting at desks, so their back muscles are out of shape and vulnerable. But good planning—wearing sunscreen to ward off ultraviolet (UV) rays and skin cancer, protecting the eyes with appropriate safety lenses, and strengthening abdominal and back muscles to avoid lower back problems—will make leisure sports as safe as they are psychologically rewarding.

# The Skin

As the body's primary protector and its single largest organ, the skin takes a beating in the gym, the pool, and out on the playing field. Friction from rubbing, the sweat from competition, and damage from sun, heat, cold, moist or dry climes, salt water, and pool chemicals can provoke a number of problems, ranging from those that are irritating to ones that require extensive medical treatment. Here are some of the more common.

## Prickly Heat (Miliaria)

Though we tend to associate prickly heat with infants, it is often a source of considerable discomfort for athletes. A condition tied to where you live, how much you normally perspire, and what gear you wear when you perform your activity, this sweat rash may be almost as unavoidable for some as it is persistent—and controlling prickly heat can prove to be a real catch-22 for anyone who sweats profusely.

Prickly heat usually takes the form of a rash of tiny red or pink pimples that affects the trunk, arms, and skin folds. When sweat ducts become plugged, trapping perspiration in the skin's dermis or epidermis layers, the ducts can become inflamed and quite itchy. Because an episode of prickly heat can last five to six weeks, it's important to avert the conditions that cause it, and if the rash does develop, to treat symptoms aggressively. If you play sports in unrelenting heat, and/or perspire a lot, try these precautions recommended by the New Zealand Dermatological Society:

• Do whatever you can to cool down and prevent further sweating: move into the shade, play in an air-conditioned environment, take frequent water dips, or some other actions.

• Wear loose-fitting clothing made of nonirritating, breathable fibers such as cotton. You may want to avoid fabrics that cling, as these can contain your body's heat and perspiration.

• Add one gram of vitamin C per day to your diet.

• Relieve itching with drying solutions like calamine lotion or a 0.5 percent hydrocortisone cream.

**SMART SOURCES**

The American Academy
   of Dermatology
PO Box 4014
Schaumburg, IL
   60168-4014
(847) 330-0230
www.aad.org

The AAD is the largest
of all dermatologic
associations with a
membership of over
11,000 dermatologists
worldwide. The AAD
offers a number of
informative brochures
at no charge.

## Athlete's foot
### (tinea pedis)

• Long thought to be highly contagious among family members, new research indicates that one family member may have athlete's foot without spreading it to anyone else.

• Another popular misconception is that you can catch the fungus by walking barefoot in the locker room.

• Women and children under 12 don't normally contract athlete's foot. If similar symptoms appear, the cause is likely to be something different.

• A rash isn't always athlete's foot, even if symptoms are similar. Because applying over-the-counter athlete's foot preparations to a nonfungal infection can be harmful, check with your doctor first.

# Athlete's Foot

Like prickly heat, athlete's foot crops up in parts of the body that are warm and moist. Unlike sweat rash, a fungus causes athlete's foot. Aptly named because athlete's foot appears more common in feet shod with sports shoes, trainers, and shoes with artificial soles, which cause the feet to sweat more heavily, the fungus causes an itchy, red, scaly rash most prevalent between the toes. Sometimes it spreads, causing cracks and bleeding in the skin.

Most common in adult males and teenagers, athlete's foot is "caused by living germs, like small plants, that grow and multiply on all humans," according to the American Academy of Dermatology (AAD). Though some people may actually have the fungus on their skin, athlete's skin won't develop unless the right conditions are present—moisture, lack of ventilation of the feet, and sweating.

To prevent athlete's foot, keep the area between the toes dry and cool. The AAD offers some additional tips:

• Always dry feet thoroughly after swimming or bathing.

• Avoid wearing tight shoes, especially in the summer.

• Wear sandals in the summertime to keep feet ventilated.

• Alternate shoes, and choose cotton over synthetics socks. Change socks frequently.

• Use an antifungal powder in shoes during the summer.

- Go barefoot at home.

A variety of over-the-counter sprays, creams, and powders containing chemicals like miconazole and clotrimazole will kill the fungus and relieve symptoms. But athlete's foot isn't necessarily over when symptoms disappear. That's why it's essential to use medications for an additional two weeks after symptoms disappear.

Sometimes the presence of athlete's foot opens the door to other marauding bacteria. If the rash seems to improve, then flare up, then improve, and on and on, see your doctor. He may prescribe foot soaks in addition to antifungal creams; for the most stubborn cases antifungal pills may be recommended.

# Jock Itch *(Tinea cruris)*

Another skin eruption—this time in the groin and upper thighs—jock itch causes painful itching as well as a scaly red rash that may leak a clear discharge. Wearing cotton underwear and applying a drying talcum powder after activities should prevent it.

# Foot Blisters

Relief for one of the most common athletic afflictions—friction blisters—may be as near as your antiperspirant. Blisters, according to the AAD, result from materials rubbing against skin that's perspired heavily.

To see if a reduction in foot perspiration might

**F.Y.I.**

• Because sunburn is caused by ultraviolet light, not heat, athletes can become burned even in cold weather.

• Skiers are at risk for sunburn because light is reflected from snow.

• Sunburn risk increases in late winter and spring.

• To prevent your nose from being burned, use zinc oxide ointment. To protect the delicate skin of the lips, use a lip balm with sunscreen.

reduce friction and consequently the formation of blisters, the academy monitored the affect of antiperspirant application to the feet of U.S. military cadets prior to a 21-kilometer hike. After comparing the results with those of a control group using a placebo preparation, the academy found that "sweat reduction was indeed a key mechanism for reducing blisters."

However, the academy also discovered that in more than half of the cadets the use of antiperspirants for five consecutive nights prior to the hike could cause an allergic reaction—itching skin and a rash.

If you're interested in trying this solution, you might avoid the allergic reaction by applying an antiperspirant on alternate nights, rather than every night, as did the cadets. You might also experiment with various preparations to find those that contain a concentration of the active ingredient aluminum chloride hexahydrate lower than the 20 percent used in the study.

# Sunburn

Swimming, running, golf, and tennis are sports in which athletes have the greatest chance of getting sunburned. According to the AAD, any tan is bad for skin, leading to wrinkling and the possibility of skin cancer 10 to 20 years later. For protection, wearing a sunscreen with at least an SPF of 15 is essential, particularly between 10 A.M. and 3 P.M. Fair-skinned, blue-eyed redheads or blonds need an even higher SPF. Golfers should consider wearing two gloves so that both hands are exposed to the same amount of sunlight, preventing premature aging of one hand due to unequal sun exposure.

It's easy to forget that the protective qualities of sunscreen can be washed off during swimming or heavy perspiration. And sun-sensitivity is heightened when you use certain deodorant soaps, perfumes, antibiotics like tetracycline, medications like Acutane and Retin-A, and some blood pressure prescriptions, further increasing the risk of developing an acute sunburn. Unless you want to look like an ad for Coppertone, stay away from sunscreens containing tropical oils like banana and coconut, which also increase sun sensitivity.

Altitude also affects how quickly you become sunburned. It also ups your risk of becoming exposed to ultraviolet light, one of the key factors in the development of skin cancer. For each 1,000 feet of elevation, ultraviolet intensity increases approximately 8 to 10 percent. That translates into about a 115 percent increase in nonmelanoma skin cancer for year-round residents living at 8,500 feet. The rate for melanoma is also higher, though exact figures are not yet available.

To put the problem in perspective, at noon on a clear day an athlete with average complexion wearing no sunscreen would burn after only six minutes of sun exposure in Vail, 11,000 feet above sea level. It would take the same person more than four times longer to become sunburned at sea level in New York, and just slightly more than two times longer to become burned in Orlando. Despite the difference in altitude, the intensity of UV light in Orlando, a site nearly 775 miles closer to the equator, is the same as in Vail. It makes good skin sense to up the SPF of the sunscreen you use if you pursue sports at high altitudes or in areas close to the equator.

**SMART DEFINITION**

**Sun Protection Factor (SPF)**

These ratings refer to the amount of sun protection a preparation offers. The higher the product's SPF, the longer a person can stay in the sun without burning, as compared to someone wearing no sun protection at all.

# Recognizing Skin Cancer

There are three types of skin cancer, each of which has its own distinguishing characteristics.

**Basal-cell carcinoma.** The most common skin cancer—comprising 80 percent of all nonmelanomas—usually appears on sun-exposed areas such as the head, face, neck, hands, and trunk. The malignancy can be as small as a pinpoint or as large as an inch and looks like a raised, translucent, pearly nodule, which may crust or bleed. It strikes one of seven Americans, but this slow-growing cancer is seldom deadly.

**Squamous-cell carcinoma.** The second most common skin cancer, these wart-like growths are also found on exposed areas. Squamous-cell cancers often look like raised pink patches with an open, oozing center. If untreated, a precancerous condition called *citini keratosis,* which appears as small and slightly raised brown, gray, or red scaly spots, can develop into this type of carcinoma. Squamous-cell cancers can spread through the bloodstream to other organs.

**Malignant melanoma.** The least common and most deadly skin cancer, melanoma is increasing faster than any other form of the disease. It strikes about twice as many men as women, possibly because men are more likely to have jobs that require them to work outdoors. Melanomas may appear suddenly on or near a mole, usually on the upper back or legs. Brown-black or multicolored with jagged borders, these malignancies may bleed or crust. Melanoma grows quickly and may spread to other organs.

# Cold-Season Dry Skin

Danger to the skin doesn't disappear when temperature drops and the sun plays hide and seek with the clouds. In fact, a skin-care regimen that would ordinarily cause few problems in summer can really dry out skin in dry, cold climates. Here's how to make the best of a potentially bad situation for your skin, courtesy of *Winter Skin Care,* published online by Gaelen Health Care:

• Because the alkaline pH in soap can dry—even burn skin—use beauty bars rather than soap.

• A moisturizing gel is less drying than soap as a base for shaving the legs.

• After shaving the legs, always use skin lotion. (You might want to try using canned hydrogenated shortening, such as Crisco, as an inexpensive but very effective alternative to commercial skin moisturizers.)

• Aftershaves that don't contain alcohol are less drying to the skin.

• Protect elbows, knees, feet, and hands where skin is thicker with a layer of moisturizer that contains alpha-hydroxy acid.

Winter climes can also pose unique challenges to those who, like Southern California athletes, live the equivalent of the eternal summer lifestyle. That's because they don't usually consider the possibility of becoming sunburned in the winter, don't remember to put on enough layers of the right clothes to keep warm, and are unfamiliar with how cool weather can harm skin.

Because lengthy hot showers, lathering up with lots of soap, and hot tub soaks can dry the skin on the face, arms, and lower legs, it's smart to spare the soap and cut the amount of hot water soak time. Drying, peeling, and itching skin are also the direct fallout from performing sports in cold,

**F.Y.I.**

The right clothing, as well as the right equipment, can help prevent dehydration, hypothermia, and respiratory problems caused by cold climates. To get you suited up appropriately, the *Georgia Tech Sports Medicine & Performance Newsletter* suggests:

• Runners and cross-country skiers should wear microfiber polyester fabrics to stay warm with fewer layers of clothing.

• In moderately cold weather, a microfiber shirt worn underneath a sweatshirt should keep your chest warm.

• Most heat escapes from the head so wear a hat!

• Because you may need to shed clothing as your body heats up in intense play, dress for the cold in layers. Bundle back up when you're not playing.

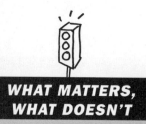

WHAT MATTERS,
WHAT DOESN'T

## What Matters

• Cleaning a wound with a 3 percent solution of hydrogen peroxide to effectively lift out dirt particles.

• Cleansing a wound by allowing it to bleed for a few seconds.

• Allowing small cuts to heal by exposure to air.

## What Doesn't

• Using alcohol on a cut or scrape because it isn't a very effective cleansing agent.

• Applying a Band-Aid to a small cut.

• Suturing small (less than one inch long) and shallow cuts (under an inch deep).

mountainous regions with low humidity or in warm, dry indoor-sports environments. Consistent use of a good moisturizer can help mitigate the effects of environmentally drying conditions.

# Other Minor Skin Injuries

Of course, not all skin problems are weather related. Many, in fact, are created by particular sporting activities.

## Black Heel/Palm

Golfers, tennis, and baseball players are prone to black heel or palm, a condition in which the injured skin becomes discolored in a spot where skin has been repeatedly pressured to slide sideways. The pressure causes tiny veins in the skin to break open and bleed into the skin. Given a chance to rest, the skin will heal naturally on its own.

## Runner's Rump

Runners and basketball players tend to develop round, purplish spots and darkened skin on the upper-middle part of the buttocks as skin rubs against itself during long periods of running. Discoloration vanishes when the amount of running is curtailed.

## Jogger's Nipples

Caused by the irritation of coarse clothing against the sensitive skin of the aureole and nipple, jogger's nipple is common in male athletes as well as women who don't wear bras while running or playing sports. Wearing shirts made of natural fibers (like cotton) and protecting the nipples with Vaseline or Band-Aids will relieve irritation.

## Minor Cuts, Abrasions, and Bruises

It's easy to suffer minor cuts, abrasions, or bruises playing leisure sports. Though these aren't usually serious, they should be treated promptly to prevent infection or other problems. And they can easily be treated on the spot. Minor cuts should be thoroughly washed with nonirritating soap and left open to the air to promote healing. Bruises that become particularly painful can be treated with an ice bag. In rare instances you may need medical attention if:

• A cut continues bleeding despite the application of pressure for 15 minutes.

• Something is embedded under the cut.

• An infection seems evident because the wound is oozing or red.

# The Hair

Blonds and fair-haired people spending many hours in a chlorine pool may experience a reverse type of alchemy as gold turns to green. Known as swimmers' hair, the greening of haircolor comes from copper ions naturally present in the water or from algaecides used for pool maintenance. To restore hair to its usual crowning glory, apply a bleaching solution of 3 percent hydrogen peroxide.

## SMART DEFINITION

**Scrape**

A common occurrence in falls from bikes or in racquet sports, a scrape is a wound in which outer layers of skin are actually scraped off. The inner skin layers or tissue underneath becomes exposed.

**Bruise**

Caused by the breakage of small blood vessels beneath the skin due to a fall or bump, the seepage of blood into surrounding tissues causes the skin to turn black and blue.

# The Head and Neck

Because of the risk of injury to the brain or the spinal column, little is more frightening than an injury to the head or neck. Much of that danger can be eliminated by wearing sports-appropriate helmets when skiing, cycling, or horseback riding.

## Head Injuries

Athletes who play leisure sports don't normally think they're at risk for a head injury because their activities don't involve body-to-body contact. That's where they're wrong. Taking a bad spill skiing, cycling, or horseback riding or getting hit in the head with a ball can also place an athlete in jeopardy. The trick is to sort out which injuries are minor and which are not.

But that's not always easy. Serious symptoms don't always show up immediately. An injured person may seem fine after a fall or another accident, but the danger of life-threatening conditions are still relevant hours later because of the nature of the many types of injuries to the brain.

To prevent such a crisis, *Active First Aid Online!* and the *Healthwise Handbook* suggest being aware of the key signs indicating an injury is serious:

• Yellowish liquid from the nose or ears. Leaks of cerebro-spinal fluid (CSF) occur when the base of the skull is fractured.

• Bruising around the eyes and behind the ears indicating the skull may have suffered a strong blow. Discoloration around the eyes doesn't necessarily indicate that the athlete has been hit in the face.

• Change in vision; objects look blurred or doubled indicating a blow to the brain. This is commonly associated with serious concussions.

• Loss of consciousness.

• Change in normal speech, confusion, memory loss.

• Weakness or numbness specific to one side of the body.

• Severe headache.

• Violent vomiting persisting beyond 15 minutes after the injury or vomiting two hours after the accident.

• Convulsions.

The best thing one can do while waiting for emergency services to arrive is to stop any severe bleeding and prevent further injury by keeping the athlete quiet. If there isn't bleeding, that does not necessarily mean the injury is minor. There could still be internal bleeding and swelling inside the skull.

Fortunately, most of the bumps to the head that occur in leisure sports will be relatively minor. While they may cause cuts that bleed profusely initially, that's generally because the scalp's blood vessels are close to the skin surface. Bleeding or not, all head injuries bear watching for the first 24 hours.

**F.Y.I.**

According to the U.S. Consumer Product Safety Commission 1999 report *Skiing Helmets: An Evaluation of the Potential to Reduce Head Injury,* a majority of injuries to the head, neck, and face in five different sports could be prevented by wearing helmets. The following statistics note the number of injuries per year to those critical areas in different sports.

• Cycling: more than a third of all injuries (about 181,000)

• Snow skiing: about 15 percent of all injuries (12,700)

• In-line skating: like skiing, about 15 percent (15,000) of the total injuries

• Mountain biking: about 18 percent (3,940) of injuries

**SMART SOURCES**

**Head Injuries and Other Information**

For more information on treating head injuries, visit the following web sites:

www.physsportsmed.com
www.parasolemt.com.

**Eye Injuries and Other Information**

The American Academy of Ophthalmology
PO Box 7424
San Francisco, CA 94120-7424
(415) 561-8500
www.eyenet.org
www.swmed.edu

Prevent Blindness America
www.preventblind-ness.org

Ninety years old in 1998, Prevent Blindness America is the nation's leading volunteer eye health and safety organization dedicated to fighting blindness and saving sight.

Even when head injuries are mild, athletes should be in no rush to return to play. According to a study by researchers at the University of North Carolina, it takes a minimum of three days for balance to return to normal after becoming hurt. Getting back into sports prematurely before an injury has had sufficient time to heal opens the door to secondary impact syndrome, a potentially fatal complication in which the brain can swell rapidly.

## Tooth Injuries

Even if you're not involved in contact sports, taking a spill or a ball in the face might result in a knocked-out tooth. If the tooth can't be reseeded on the spot, you'll need to preserve it carefully until you reach the dentist's office. Don't try to scrape dirt off the tooth; just rinse it in salt water or milk, if available. Milk is also a great medium in which to place the tooth while it's transported to the dentist; if milk isn't available, place it between your cheek and teeth.

## Eye Injuries

The good news about eye injuries is that more than 90 percent of them could be prevented if people wore sports-specific guards, glasses, and shields. That is particularly true for those at high risk of injury—beginning athletes with low skill levels; and people with pre-existing eye conditions, high prescriptions, and those who've had eye surgery.

"If one is playing with low vision in one eye and good vision in another, precautions should be taken to protect the good eye," the National Society to Prevent Blindness points out. "Otherwise, an injury could reduce the athlete's overall vision. Due to the inherent weaknesses pre-existing in their eyes, people who have high prescriptions might be at a bigger risk for permanent damage. The same applies to those who've had eye surgery because it may have weakened the natural state of the eye."

Young players under the age of 25 are at very high risk; three out of four eye injuries occur in this age group.

## Protecting the Eyes from UV Rays

If you're going to engage in outdoor sports, you'll need to wear sunglasses with adequate protection against ultraviolet light. When buying sunglasses,

**F.Y.I.**

The National Society to Prevent Blindness estimates the total number of eye injuries related to sports and recreation to be close to 100,000. Eye injuries often result in permanent damage, yet most people do not take any measures to protect their eyes.

# Buying Sports Eye Protectors

• If you wear glasses, your eye doctor can fit you with prescription eyeguards.

• Buy eyeguards containing lenses at optical or sports stores. To protect the eye in case of an accident, these lenses should either "pop outward or stay in place." Never purchase any that pop in against the eyes.

• To protect against fogging lenses, look for eyeguards with antifog protective coatings or side vents.

• Make sure the products have been tested for application to sports and that they're made of impact resistant polycarbonate material.

• To minimize the possibility of cuts from the eyeguards, buy those that are padded along the brow and nose bridge.

*Source:* Prevent Blindness America

the American Academy of Ophthalmology recommends those that have been tested to protect eyes against UV 400. Expect the protection to come with a higher price tag: most inexpensive sunglasses do not cover this range, so you may have to spend a little more.

## Treating Minor Eye Injuries

Wearing the right protective eye gear will minimize your chances of getting injured. But if something minor does happen to your eye, some easy first aid should get the problem under control. If a foreign object does strike or attach to your eye, don't try to dislodge it by pushing it around in your eye or by using eye drops unless your doctor instructs you to do so.

Before attempting to treat your eye, wash your hands. Then gently bathe a bloodshot or irritated eye with cool water. If something is lodged in the side of the eye or on the lower lid, try to remove it with a moist cotton swab. Don't rub it and do not use tweezers or similar objects to remove it.

## Treating Major Eye Injuries

Persistent or severe pain, blurred vision that does not correct after something's been removed from the eye, a foreign object adhered to the pupil or the white of the eye, or a puncture all need emergency care. The best you can do until a doctor examines the eye is to close your eyes, if possible, and keep them covered.

# Neck Injuries

Although the incidence of a catastrophic neck injury is low in most leisure sports, athletes participating in diving and equestrian events are at increased risk. "Another group of athletes with very distinct physical symptoms is also at risk for neurologic problems that cannot be detected with routine physicals," say the Charlotte Orthopedic Specialists. "These people almost always have warning signs while participating in athletics. Such warning signs include 'burners' or 'stingers' involving pain and/or numbness radiating down both arms simultaneously. The isolated burner or stinger that involves only one upper extremity at a time and disappears with rest is another story. These symptoms don't predispose the athlete to an increased risk of catastrophic neck injury, but they should be discussed with a physician."

If you participate in sports in which falling is a risk, you ought to be able to recognize the symptoms of whiplash (neck strain) and understand how to treat it.

When an athlete falls and the neck is forced into an extreme position, stretching or tearing ligaments connecting the vertebrae, the first indication that he may have suffered a neck sprain is a sharp pain on one side of the neck. Though the pain might dissipate after an hour or so, it can often return as a dull ache followed by acute pain. Moving the head may be difficult because of neck muscle spasms, headache, and even dizziness.

Over-the-counter pain medications and ice for two to three days applied in customary first-aid fashion will reduce pain and swelling, but one should also get an evaluation from a physician to rule out serious injuries.

Once the pain has gone and a physician has signed off on the presence of any extensive injuries, you then may begin a program of range-of-motion exercises, under your doctor's approval. The idea is to move the head in four different directions.

After full range of motion has been restored and the neck is free of pain and spasms and almost back to its normal strength, the athlete can return to play.

# The Back

Every year, 50 percent of working-age Americans suffer a "back attack." Seventy-five percent of the time backs go out when sitters attempt to instantly transform themselves into athletes after working hours. Overweight, out of condition, in a hurry to play like a pro without taking the time to master form or strengthen abdominal muscles, the weekend athlete is at high risk for back injury.

## Back Injuries

Second only to the common cold in frequency of visits to the doctor, some 20 million American suffer back injuries every year. The bill for medical treatment and lost time at work exceeds $30 billion.

About 95 percent of all back attacks are the result of being in poor physical condition. A number of other factors can up your chance of developing a back problem after age 30:

• Your job requires sitting most of the day or conversely, heavy manual labor.

• You have poor posture, lean forward for extended periods, or use office furniture that isn't ergonomically sound.

• You smoke. (Smoking may interfere with blood circulation to the disk.)

• You're stressed.

• You play sports involving lots of twisting or high impact.

The good news is that up to 90 percent of backaches get better on their own within one month.

## Back Spasms

The most common type of backache is a sudden, violent spasm of muscles resulting from a trauma to a muscle or disk. Athletes at high risk for muscle spasms are those who "move primarily in one direction because that one repetitive motion can result in trauma," physical therapist Don Van Volkenburg, P.T., C.S.C.S, who treats athletes at the Peachtree Orthopaedic Clinic in Atlanta told the *Penn State Sports Medicine Newsletter.* "The other type of high risk athlete is the weekend warrior who does not exercise during the week, then overdoes it on the weekend."

What can sometimes happen is that the muscle tightness triggered by a long-lasting spasm can cause more muscle contractions. Positions in which you bend forward or are in between sitting

**SMART SOURCES**

The American Chiropractic Association
1701 Clarendon Blvd.
Arlington, VA 22209
(800) 986-4636

The ACA can provide brochures on back pain and a list of chiropractors in your area.

and standing seem most likely to trigger additional spasms, the *Newsletter* points out.

The cure is to stop the activity that initiated the pain, but try to stay out of bed. Not long ago, up to two weeks of bed rest was recommended; now doctors advise keeping that down to a maximum of two days. Those who stay as active as they can, even if they have some pain, get better faster than those who remain sedentary. Control pain with aspirin, ibuprofen, acetaminophen, or nonsteroidal anti-inflammatory drugs, rather than muscle relaxants, which make 30 percent of patients sleepy.

For the first 48 to 72 hours, use ice, not heat, even if no swelling is apparent. "Because ice decreases blood flow and numbs the painful area, it's better than heat, which prolongs inflammation by bringing too much blood flow in," says Van Volkenburg.

For acute low back pain lasting more than two weeks, a 1996 study by the Agency for Health Care Policy and Research reports that a short course of manipulation by a chiropractor or osteopath is more effective than forms of routine care. Relief should occur within 6 to 12 treatments; if not, see your family doctor.

The agency suggests you think twice before trying ultrasound, traction, support belts, massage, biofeedback, acupuncture, or any injections for acute back pain within the first month. Their advice is to allow the body to heal itself without rushing into expensive diagnostic tests or, especially, surgery.

If you develop sciatica (pain that radiates down your leg from your lower back), experts on the agency panel recommend an X-ray and a focused assessment of your medical history to rule out any undiagnosed problems before any manipulation.

# Getting the Back into Shape

Just because you've had an episode of backache or have some of the risk factors doesn't mean sports are out of the question. However, it does indicate you should begin a conditioning program to strengthen abdominal and extensor muscles in the back that support the spinal column along with developing flexibility in the hamstrings and lower back. Many of the sports that pose little or no risk of injury—like swimming, biking, hiking, cross-country skiing, race walking, and skating—are also great for overall conditioning.

But even these can be made more back friendly with the right equipment and attention to form:

• **Race walking:** Buy a pair of sports shoes designed to absorb shock.

• **Swimming:** Breathing through a snorkel will make twisting the neck to take a breath above the water unnecessary. Instead of the butterfly stroke (absolutely off-limits for back pain sufferers) or the breast and Australian crawl, do the side or backstroke.

• **Cycling:** Modify handlebars or buy a mountain bike for a more upright posture so there's less pressure on your back. Avoid models like racing bikes that cause you to crouch forward.

## Your Sport May Not Be the Culprit . . .

Just because your lower back began aching after participating in a sport, don't necessarily assume the sport's to blame. New Zealand physical thera-

## STREET SMARTS

By any measure, elementary school-teacher Robin Radlauer, 45, is an avid athlete. But a motorcycle accident she had could have sharply curtailed her athletic life. "I'd just gotten off the bike and put the kickstand down," she says. "But I didn't secure it correctly, and the bike started to fall toward me, forcing me to catch it. I managed to prevent it from landing on me, but in doing so I really sprained my back."

Since this was Robin's second back injury, the chiropractor treating her recommended a series of back-strengthening exercises. "I spend about 30 minutes a day doing these before leaving for school, and I get an adjustment monthly," she says. "Thanks to this routine, I'm in good back health and still very active in sports!"

pist Robin McKenzie, O.B.E., F.C.S.P., author of *Treat Your Own Back,* points out that your posture after the game is over may actually be at fault: "Most people sit down and collapse in a heap. Slouching like this, which puts the spine in extreme positions, can cause the soreness."

To see if this applies to you, McKenzie suggests sorting out the timing of pain—did it begin during or after play? If it commenced while you were playing, he suggests relief may be found by performing a series of standing back extensions. With knees straight and hands in the small of the back, slowly arc your trunk backward.

Don't be surprised if the pain isn't timed to the exercise itself; McKenzie points out that 60 percent of exercisers may have faulty postexercise posture. He suggests that athletes may short-circuit back pain by paying particular attention to sitting correctly after playing by using a lumbar support pillow in the small of the back. He also recommends that athletes watch their posture as they're waiting for their turn at golf, tennis, track and field, and others.

## The Way to a Healthy Back: Stretch and Exercise

One of the best ways to prevent low back pain is through a thorough program of stretching. The *Georgia Tech Sports Medicine & Performance Newsletter* recommends four stretches:

• **The bent-knee crunch**, in which you lie down, with feet flat on floor, knees bent, and arms crossed on chest, and raise your head and shoulders about

30 degrees; hold for five seconds. Begin with one to three crunches and increase the repetitions as you become stronger.

• **The pelvic tilt** is an isometric exercise performed with your back on the floor and knees bent. Tighten your lower abdominal muscles and buttocks, holding for 10 seconds, relax, and repeat three times.

• **The lower back stretch** is performed sitting on the floor with legs extended. Reach forward toward your toes and hold the stretch for 10 seconds, repeating three times. Try to increase the stretch with subsequent exercises.

• **The knees-to-chest stretch** is performed lying on the floor, bringing both knees to the chest and holding them with your arms and hands for 10 seconds. Return to the starting position with both legs on the floor. Then repeat the exercise bringing just the left knee to the chest, holding for 10 seconds. Next, bring both knees to the chest, followed by just the right knee. Do this cycle in the morning and before retiring at night.

You may also want to consider tumbling, rolling on the ground, even hanging upside down on a jungle gym as a preventive measure to keep the spine supple and the body in balance. That's the advice of Philip Santiago, D.C., a sports chiropractor and former professional soccer player who now counsels Olympic athletes and amateurs. "Kids don't hurt their backs very often because they roll around and tumble and do acrobatics," he points out. "They're maintaining their body computers, staying in balance."

## THE BOTTOM LINE

Though playing sports is great, being physically active poses unique risks. Summer heat can cause a variety of uncomfortable skin conditions, along with sunburn and skin cancer. Sports like golf, tennis, running, and basketball, in which skin is under constant stress, can cause transient problems.

Getting hit with a ball may cause injury to the eyes unless the athlete is wearing proper eye protection. Necks can be strained and backs can spasm, but exercises designed to strengthen the abdominal muscles and others in the back supporting the spine can go a long way toward conditioning the body to withstand the challenges of sports gracefully and painlessly.

Santiago also suggests conditioning the back muscles and improving balance by using an exercise ball or balance beam, rowing, or doing squats as you walk. He even has golfers get conditioned by standing on a balance beam, heels hanging off one side. Then they work to swing the club straight without falling off.

To be successful playing sports, the athlete needs more than just good eyesight, agility, coordination, and strong muscles. Needed also are a considerable dose of common sense and the smarts to take the extra time to fit, buy, and put on protective gear such as a helmet, eyewear, and sunscreen—all necessary to prevent an afternoon of playing sports from turning into a medical crisis. But even athletes with good equipment may suffer the unexpected accident. Knowing what to do if there's a minor injury and what merits immediate medical attention are equally essential elements to playing well and intelligently.

......................

# Treating Common Injuries: Shoulder to Hand

For athletes who become addicted to their game, the old adage "Use it or lose it" really ought to be "Overuse it and lose it." Nowhere does that apply more than to the structures integral to the arm and hand. So much of the pain recreational athletes experience could be avoided by proper conditioning and strengthening, attention to form and equipment, and the smarts to know when a pain signal is really the body's way of calling 911.

# The Shoulder

All it takes is a tumble onto an outstretched arm while you're skating, biking, or skiing to cause an injury to your shoulders. While such accidents are unpredictable, wearing shoulder pads and learning how to fall can minimize chances of becoming seriously injured. Regardless of which sport you play, train yourself to avoid falling on a shoulder or outstretched arm. Instead, try to tuck arms in and roll over onto your trunk to minimize injuries.

## Collarbone Dislocations and Separations

The most common injuries to the shoulder area are often to the collarbone, which can suffer dislocations or separations.

If you do fall directly on the top of the shoulder, you probably will separate or dislocate the acromioclavicular (AC) joint between the collarbone (clavicle) and the shoulder, spraining or tearing the ligaments holding the collarbone in place. The seriousness of the injury depends on whether you've sprained or actually torn the ligaments. If the injury is just a sprain (classified as a Grade I or II), all you'll need for healing is to wear a sling for a few weeks to control pain. But if the collarbone is elevated and there's a pronounced bump on top of the shoulder, a complete tear of the ligaments (called a Grade III) has probably occurred. While the collarbone is likely to always remain elevated, 90 percent of those who incur this injury are able to resume normal activities once the clavicle heals. Whether or not surgery should be undertaken to repair the torn ligaments and relocate the AC joint in very severe Grade III injuries is controversial, and is usually reserved mainly for professional athletes whose careers are at stake. Most of the time, conservative treatment such as immobilizing the joint by putting the arm into a sling will suffice.

## Collarbone Fractures

A fall might have a more serious outcome, resulting in a fracture—a cracking, breaking, or complete shattering of the collarbone. Symptoms include swelling and tenderness in the area, discoloration, inability to move the shoulder, and the sound of crunching from the broken bones. After emergency first aid—splinting your arm to your body, putting it in a sling, and applying ice—get it to an emergency room. While surgery is probably a remote possibility, recovery will likely involve wearing the arm in a sling for a few weeks (if the collarbone isn't broken) or wearing a brace for six weeks or more if it is.

**SMART DEFINITION**

**Grades of sprains and strains**

Strains and sprains are graded according to the severity of symptoms and the percentage of fibers that are stretched, torn, or completely ruptured.

**Grade I** is the most mild injury, involving damage to less than 25 percent of fibers.

**Grade II** involves tearing between 25 to 75 percent of the fibers.

**Grade III** is a complete rupture.

Here's some good advice on transporting a person with an injured shoulder to the emergency room:

### Dislocations

If the dislocated joint has been immobilized, position the person in the vehicle so that the area remains stationary. Do not try to fix the dislocation yourself. Incorrectly pulling or manipulating a bone can cause nerve and blood vessel injury.

### Sprains

Continue the ice, elevation, and compression that were administered during first aid. Keep the joint immobile.

*Source:* Earl Grubbs, M.D., *Penn State Sports Medicine Newsletter*

# Acromioclavicular (AC) Joint Injuries

Sometimes a spill will separate the joint where the end of the collarbone meets the shoulder blade, thrusting the collarbone out of alignment. The seriousness of the injury depends on how much pain and swelling there is and whether or not the outer edge of the collarbone sticks up. Use the RICE technique (see page 32) for the injury, applying ice 20 minutes on and 20 minutes off as frequently as possible for the first 10 days and keep the arm in a sling. If you can't move your shoulder or raise your arm over your head, and the shoulder remains painful 10 days later, see a doctor. If you have suffered a severe Grade III separation, the shoulder will require immobilization for six weeks as well as physical rehabilitation.

# Shoulder Dislocation

If the shape of the shoulder changes as the result of a fall so that the outside suddenly looks flat rather than round and movement causes excruciating pain, you've probably dislocated the shoulder. Apply first aid and the RICE technique, and put your arm in a sling or splint it to the body. Do not attempt to realign the dislocation if you aren't medically trained. That requires the skills of a physician who will relocate the shoulder under anesthetic. Afterward, wearing the arm in a sling for about three weeks will allow the ligaments and capsule to heal.

# Overuse Injuries

Excessive overhead motion, such as throwing a baseball, spiking a volleyball, serving in tennis, or the butterfly stroke in swimming, may trigger overuse injuries in which the rotator cuff muscles holding the shoulder bones in place are stretched. Trying to gain more rotation in the shoulder for greater speed in throwing or serving can make matters worse, so that the simple motion of lifting your arm overhead becomes difficult.

The most important part of getting better is to rest the shoulder by avoiding the sport that caused the problem. But rest in itself is only part of the cure. To prevent reoccurrence, the rotator cuff muscles will need to be strengthened and some of the ways in which you perform a sport revamped.

First, you'll need to reduce the pain and inflammation using an over-the-counter medication like aspirin and by applying the RICE formula.

Whatever you do, don't give into the temptation to "baby" your shoulder by not moving it at all. This will cause you to develop a secondary problem—frozen shoulder. That just leads to the formation of adhesions causing ligaments in the shoulder to stick together. Be sure to perform range of motion exercises throughout the day to maintain flexibility.

## Tendinitis and Bursitis

Common overuse injuries develop when the tendons holding the ball of the shoulder in place or when the fluid-filled bursa between the tendons and the shoulder blade have become inflamed. These conditions, tendinitis and bursitis respectively, are treated in the same manner as other overuse injuries.

**STREET SMARTS**

Anne Este, 35, is an admitted tennis addict. She loves the game so much that on occasion she will play through pain, hoping it will disappear. Last spring, she was playing the finals at her club. But every time she served, her shoulder hurt. She was so close to the title she just kept pushing. In the last game, she felt something pop. Thomas Wickiewicz, M.D., chief of sports medicine at the Hospital for Special Surgery in New York City, examined her and delivered the bad news. She had torn her rotator cuff and would require surgery. "It's so sad," she says. "If I'd stopped and consulted the doctor when the pain first started, my shoulder could have been treated with RICE, a sling, and physical therapy. Now I need surgery!"

## SMART DEFINITION

**Tendon**

Tough ropelike cord that connects muscle to bone or other tissue.

**Tendinitis**

Tenderness of the tendon or surrounding tissues, resulting from injury, overuse, and movements that require repeated twisting or rapid joint movement. Splitting and tearing of tendons may result from an acute injury like a fall.

**Bursa**

Fluid-filled sacs that help muscles slide easily over other muscles or bones.

**Bursitis**

Inflammation of the bursa, caused by overuse of a joint or tendon, resulting in pain and redness. The condition can occur at several different places throughout the body and can appear in conjunction with tendinitis.

A tip off that shoulder pain is the result of tendinitis or bursitis is its location. According to the *Healthwise Handbook*: "Shoulder pain on the outside of the upper arm is often due to tendinitis or bursitis in the shoulder joint. But pain on the top of the shoulder or in the neck is often due to tension in the trapezius muscles, which run from the back of the head across the back of the shoulders."

If RICE doesn't relieve the pain, you could be a candidate for an injection of a steroid, such as cortisone. Arthroscopic surgery to remove the inflamed tissue and create more space for the irritated tendons is a last resort. Conventional "open" surgery may be required to repair tears in the rotator cuff.

To prevent developing bursitis or tendinitis, try these strengthening exercises for the rotator cuff muscles recommended by the American Academy of Orthopaedic Surgeons:

• **Basic Shoulder Strengthening:** Attach elastic tubing to a doorknob. Gently pull the tubing toward your body. Hold for a count of five. Repeat five times with each arm twice a day.

• **Wall Push-Up:** Stand facing a wall with your hands on the wall and feet shoulder-width apart. Slowly perform a standing push-up, holding for a count of five. Repeat five times twice daily.

• **Shoulder Press-Up:** With your feet on the floor, sit upright on a chair with armrests. Use your arms to slowly rise off the chair, holding for a count of five. Repeat five times twice daily.

Making alterations in how you perform certain sports activities can go a long way to preventing overuse injuries. For example, when serving a tennis ball or spiking volleyball, prevent a shoulder injury by bending your trunk sideways. "Bending keeps the shoulder in a position that is less vulnerable to injury," says the *Georgia Tech Sports Medicine & Performance Newsletter.*

# The Elbow

Whether you play racquetball, squash, tennis, or golf, excessive, repetitive motion, weak muscles, and incorrect form could put you at risk to develop tennis or golf elbow—an inflammation of the tendon fibers that attach the forearm muscles to the outside of the elbow. When these tendons and muscles become inflamed, pain can become so acute that you flinch just lifting or grasping something. The pain may be experienced from the upper arm and elbow all the way down to the thumb, the domino effect of weak muscles in the upper back. Pain is generally felt during or after playing.

Among tennis players, injury appears to be a function of skill—specifically how good your backhand form actually is. "One cause of tennis elbow at every ability level is thinking of the backhand as strictly an upper body movement instead of one that incorporates the muscles of the feet, legs, hips, shoulders, arms, and hands," says the *Penn State Sports Medicine Newsletter.* "The kinetic chain is as important in hitting a backhand as in pitching a baseball."

An obvious mistake in backhand form leading to tennis elbow is to lead the stroke with the elbow, so that too much stress is put on the wrist and fore-

**SMART MOVE**

"Most recreational athletes start to experience shoulder pain because of repetitive movements or incorrect form," says Steven N. Copp, M.D., associate head of orthopedics at Scripps Clinic in La Jolla, California. "If they've only irritated the rotator cuff, applying RICE and using good judgment about how much throwing they do will resolve the problem. But if the pain is due to an underlying instability in the shoulder, the symptoms will reoccur and require more expert medical attention."

arm. This overuse leads to tennis elbow, the *Newsletter* points out. To correct the technique and reduce risk of developing tennis elbow, alter the grip on the racquet so that the inside of the thumb, rather than the bottom part, is in contact with the racquet handle.

Repositioning the role of the elbow in hitting the backhand is also advised. A change in form so that the elbow drops down, away from the body, will help but is often beyond the strength of all but advanced players. Therefore, the *Newsletter* suggests that less skilled players use a two-handed backhand. When the athlete steps into the ball, his hips rotate, causing the trunk and arms to move together. Since no movement occurs at the elbow or the wrists, less stress is placed on those two areas. And some studies have shown that players who use a one-hand backhand are twice as likely to develop tennis elbow as those who use both hands.

For golfers, elbows can also be their metaphoric Achilles' heel. Though tennis and golfer's elbows are treated similarly, the main difference is where pain is located. Due to the pulling action of the left arm as it strikes the ground with force, tenderness is generally experienced in the left inner elbow radiating down the outside of the forearm toward the pinkie. (The fact that most golfers experience pain in the left elbow is related to the large preponderance of right-handed golfers.) The cause, says the American Orthopaedic Society for Sports Medicine (AOSSM), is poor swing mechanics and conditioning.

As classic examples of tendinitis, both tennis and golfer's elbows should be treated with RICE and over-the-counter analgesics to reduce the pain and inflammation. While there's some controversy over using a strap to support the elbow during rehab because some experts feel its use can lead to other problems, there is unanimous agreement about the need for strengthening exercises.

Wait a good three days to begin these rehab exercises. "Keeping Tennis Elbow at Arm's Length" (from *The Physician and SportsMedicine)* suggests performing strengthening exercises either with a thick rubber band and tennis ball or light free weights. If you opt for the weights, be sure to warm up with five minutes of light exercise or apply a heating pad to the elbow. Sitting in a chair with your forearm resting on a table or your thigh, perform a set of 10 to 15 wrist curls using only your arm for resistance. Begin with your palm facing toward your body, and slowly bend your wrist up, flexing it to its maximum and holding for two seconds. Then reverse the exercise so that your palm faces down and you bring your wrist up toward your arm. Gradually work up to two sets of 30 repetitions. Once you can manage these exercises without pain, try working with a one pound weight for 10 reps, building up over time to 30 reps. Progress gradually to using heavier three pound weights, then move to five and eventually to seven pounds. Even though you're using more weight, keep your elbow straight (not locked) and perform a set of 20 reps without supporting your arm on a table or your thigh.

"Keeping Tennis Elbow" also outlines a series of forearm rotation exercises. Sitting with your palm up and elbow on your thigh or a table, grasp the dumbbell by one end and slowly turn the forearm until the back of your hand faces down. After maintaining the stretch for two seconds, gradually return to the original position. Follow the same progression in terms of adding weights and increasing repetitions as in the wrist curl exercises.

## SMART SOURCES

The American Academy
  of Orthopaedic
  Surgeons
PO Box 2058
Des Plaines, IL 60017
(847) 384-4138
www.aaos.org

For a free brochure about shoulder injuries, send a stamped, self-addressed envelope to *Shoulder Pain* at the above address.

The Rothman Institute
  at Jefferson Hospital
925 Chestnut Street
Philadelphia, PA
  19107-4216
(215) 955-3458
www.rothmaninstitute.
  com/sportsmed

This orthopedic center is a good source of information. Contact them directly or on the Web.

# Referred Pain: When It Hurts Somewhere Else

Even though you may occasionally experience a pain in one part of your body the actual problem may lie with an internal organ elsewhere. According to the *Penn State Sports Medicine Newsletter,* that can happen "because the painful area is served by nerves from the same part of the spinal cord as the organ. For example, a problem with the heart may cause discomfort in the neck, back, shoulders, or arms." Here's what to look for:

| Pain Source | Location of Referred Pain |
| --- | --- |
| Liver, gallbladder | Right side of neck, chest, right shoulder blade |
| Abdomen | Upper back, chest, right shoulder |
| Kidney | Back (below the ribs), groin |
| Heart | Neck, jaws, arms, shoulders, upper back |
| Lungs | Chest, jaws, neck, back |
| Teeth, gums | Ears (earache) |
| Eyes | Head (headache) |

Never exercise through pain, and modify any exercise that hurts. After each exercise session, ice the elbow for at least 10 minutes.

To see if faulty form or equipment causes part of the problem, have the grip on your golf club or racquet evaluated by a pro. When you're back on the links, make it a part of your routine to increase blood flow and flexibility in the shoulder by stretching the muscles. Don't forget to rotate your neck from side to side, stretch by touching your toes and limber up the trunk with sideways bends.

# The Wrist

With 27 bones, the wrist is a marvel of flexibility and strength. But sports put it under extreme stress. Falling wrong; catching, intercepting, or throwing a ball incorrectly; as well as poor playing technique makes the wrist highly vulnerable to strain and injury.

## Golfer's Wrist

As elsewhere in the body, repetitive motion like swinging a club or delivering an impact with a racquet can really wreak havoc in the wrist, leading to a fracture called golfer's wrist. What happens is that the hook on the hamate bone between the ring finger and pinkie gets fractured, causing considerable pain in the wrist. Despite the break, the fracture only shows up on an MRI, not X-ray, according to an interview with John F. Feller, M.D., assistant professor of radiology at Stanford University, published in the *Penn State Sports Medicine Newsletter*. In addition to wrist pain, tenderness is often felt around the pinkie side of the hand, along with numbness and difficulty in gripping.

To short-circuit the development of chronic pain, it's essential to diagnose this type of fracture early. Because there isn't much blood supply to the area, the break won't normally heal by immobilization and will probably require surgery to remove the broken hook. After surgery, strengthening exercises for the hand, fingers, and forearm are prescribed. Recovery is slow, often taking 4 to 12 weeks before the athlete can play again.

If you engage in sports with a high risk of

**SMART MOVE**

"An injury caused by moving the body the wrong way over a period of time presents athletes with two problems," says the *Penn State Sports Medicine Newsletter*. "First they have to recover from the injury. Then they have to retrain themselves so that it won't happen again."

**SMART DEFINITION**

Sometimes it's hard to tell the difference between a sprain and a strain. Here's how the American Orthopaedic Society for Sports Medicine briefly summarizes each:

**Sprain**

These involve an injury to a ligament.

**Strain**

These involve an injury to a muscle or tendon.

**SMART SOURCES**

The American Society of the Hand
6300 North River Road
Suite 600
Rosemont, IL 60018-4256
(847) 384-8300

This society publishes the free brochure "Hand Fractures."

falling, such as skiing, cycling, or skating, you are at risk for fracturing, dislocating, or spraining the wrist or fingers. According to the Consumer Product Safety Commission, while skaters wear knee and elbow pads, their wrists remain vulnerable and unprotected. Because skaters reach out automatically with their hands to break a fall, about 25 percent of all skating injuries involve injuries to the wrist. Too often athletes frequently write off accidents to the wrist as mere strains, ignoring the possibility of a fracture. Waiting weeks to obtain a proper diagnosis and medical care often sets recuperation back significantly.

## Wrist Strain from Overuse

Skiers who plant their poles in deep snow, racquet sport athletes, rowers, and canoeists often develop wrist tendinitis from backward flexing of the hand. Tenderness on the back of the forearm, swelling, and complaining tendons that squeak when the arm is moved are common symptoms. Apply the standard treatment for tendinitis—RICE along with over-the-counter analgesics to reduce pain and swelling. If this doesn't resolve the problem, you may want to try icing, cortisone injections, and splinting. When the skier returns to the slopes, he may want to switch to a shorter pole.

## Wrist Ganglion

A hard lump over a tendon in the wrist that hurts when it's pressed, plus discomfort in flexing the wrist and hand, indicates a wrist ganglion. A com-

# Choosing the Right Form of Ice Therapy

Ice is one of the most important elements in delivering first aid. To help you make the most appropriate selection to treat an injury, here's a rundown of the most common options available.

• **Gel Packs:** The advantage to these is that they can be stored in the freezer and frozen and refrozen because they contain a special gel. Since the gel remains flexible even when frozen, it contours to the injured body part. The downside is that it cools the skin faster than ice bags, requiring greater caution in application.

• **Chemical Cold Bags:** These work well in emergency situations because they need no special refrigeration as the cold effect is produced when the bag is squeezed. However, the cold produced by the chemical reaction is not particularly great, though it is helpful in first aid.

• **Immersion:** If an athlete can tolerate it, placing the injured part in frigid ice-filled water for 10 to 20 minutes is very effective.

• **Ice Massage:** Fill a paper or foam cup with water and freeze it. Strip away the upper half of the cup; the bottom of the cup can now be held and the ice used as a massager for an injury. Apply it to bony areas for no more than 10 minutes; fattier sites like the thighs can tolerate the massage for up to 20 minutes. The downside of the treatment is that the cold doesn't last as long or penetrate as deeply as other methods.

mon occurrence among bowlers and players of racquet and handball who have poor muscle strength and don't sufficiently warm up, a ganglion is generally treated with cortisone injections. If the ganglion continues to form after injections, causing pain with movement, it will have to be surgically removed.

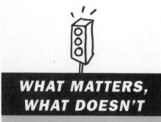

**What Matters**

• If something starts to hurt when playing, make it a point to stop the activity if the pain doesn't abate or if it gets worse.

• Skipping a few days of play might do your body a world of good if you're fighting an infection.

• If you actually do fracture your hand, be sure to maintain gentle motion while it's healing.

**What Doesn't**

• Finishing a run, a game, or a ride when pain persists and gets worse.

• Getting back into the game prematurely; if you do, a fracture or sprain might not have sufficient time to heal.

• The absence of blood: this does not mean an injury is necessarily minor.

# The Hand

Sports that involve constant gripping (rowing, golf, tennis, squash, or racquetball) can pull, strain, and even tear muscles or tendons in the hand. What you'll feel is cramping, muscle spasm, and pain with stretching and swelling. If this is a first-time injury and you don't aggravate the condition by returning to play too quickly, you might get symptoms under control with RICE and a continuing care program of ice massage for 15 minutes 4 times a day. If pain responds to heat, try using heat lamps, hot showers, or other similar applications after the first 24 hours.

## Handlebar Palsy

Though biking is one of the best sports for overall conditioning, enthusiasts who cycle long distances with a death-defying grip on the handlebars can develop handlebar palsy. A seemingly baffling set of symptoms involving numbness, tingling, and weakness of the hands, the problem is ultimately traced to an irritated nerve on the outside base of the little finger. Symptoms clear up with decreased time on the bike and a change in hand positions. Cyclists must also remember to keep their elbows loose, not locked.

# The Fingers

It's easy to sprain a finger playing sports involving striking, defending, and throwing just as it is in try-

# Sports When You're Sick?

Whether or not to keep that date for doubles or your step aerobics class can be a tough call when you're sick. Your spirit is willing, but is your body? Just how smart is pushing it—will playing make a cold, stomach flu, or other illness worse?

The answer may surprise you. William A. Primos Jr., M.D., a charter member of the American Medical Society for Sports Medicine, wrote in the article "Exercising—Or Not—When You're Sick" (published online by the McGraw-Hill Companies): "Working out can sometimes temporarily clear a stuffed-up head when you have a cold." To help you decide on the right course of action or nonaction, he suggests doing a "neck check of symptoms. If your symptoms are located 'above the neck'—a stuffy or runny nose, sneezing, or a sore throat, then exercise is probably safe. But start at half speed, increasing to full speed after 10 minutes if you're feeling okay."

Primos warns against playing sports if you are suffering from "below-the-neck symptoms, like muscle aches, hacking cough, fever over 100, chills, diarrhea, or vomiting. Otherwise, exertion may cause weakness and dehydration, even heat stroke or heart failure!"

When the acute symptoms have disappeared, he suggests "easing back into sports by playing at lower intensity for each day you were sick." To protect against spreading your cold to other players, Primos warns against sharing water bottles and towels.

ing to break a fall with an outstretched hand. Bending a finger beyond the normal range of motion or taking a hit on the fingertip also leads to sprains. The symptoms involved—pain, swelling, and inability to move the finger—will leave little doubt as to what's happened.

Whatever you do, don't tough it out by continuing to play. That can lead to a host of complications, including delayed healing and even loss of function. Treat the finger immediately with RICE.

Whether it's your toe, shoulder, wrist, or elbow that hurts, of equal concern is knowing when it's time to quit and when it's okay to continue playing. Key to making a wise decision is whether the pain gets worse or abates as you play. Getting back into the game prematurely before fractures or sprains have adequate time to heal can just make matters worse. The disappearance of symptoms is only part of the rehabilitation process. The rest is learning to correct mistakes in form or technique that may have precipitated the injury.

If you're sick, and wondering if it's okay to play, first pay attention to your symptoms and where they are. If they're above the neck, it's probably safe; below, perhaps time off is the better answer.

If you think all you have is a mild sprain, you can treat it yourself by splinting it to another finger. But if you're still symptomatic beyond two weeks, see a doctor.

# The Thumb

Downhill skiers who fall and get their thumbs caught in their pole straps may wind up with a serious injury, according to the Loyola University Health System. If the thumb is forced backward, the ligaments connecting the long bone of the thumb to the first small bone of the thumb may be stretched, torn, or completely ruptured. The university's online article "Hand Injuries" suggests immobilizing the hand and icing the injury for up to 30 minutes intermittently for 48 to 72 hours. If the pain is extreme, and the finger is very swollen or deformed, see a physician.

# Know the Signs

The key to preventing an accident from developing into a catastrophe is to pay attention to two key signs—pain and swelling. One of the first things athletes should learn is to distinguish between soreness and a sharp pain emanating from a joint and the difference between transient puffiness and swelling. Playing through pain is a sure way to play yourself out of the game.

# Treating Common Injuries: Pelvis to Foot

You can't do sports standing still, so how well your hips rotate, your knees bend, and your feet absorb the shock of running and jumping are key to how well and how safely you'll play. Paying attention to the fit of your sports shoes and even how they're laced can actually prevent many injuries, relieve pain, and give you that competitive edge.

# Body Sounds

Your body has a language all its own to communicate that an injury has occurred. For example, an Achilles tendon rupturing often feels as if you've been hit just above your heel, and the noise sounds like "a muted rifle shot." That's how Cleveland orthopedic surgeon, Angela Smith, M.D., described her own experience. The sound of a tearing ligament is also distinctive and is akin to a crackling sound.

Noises that indicate an injury has occurred are different than crepitus, the way an athlete's body sometimes creaks, cracks, and groans like an old house. While these noises ebb and wane during play, persistent noise accompanied by pain alerts you that something's gone wrong with your musculoskeletal frame.

Tendinitis, for example, often generates sound. When the tendons running from the muscles of the lower leg to the top of the foot become inflamed, you may hear a creaking noise when you flex your toes, especially in running.

A condition known as "talking ankles" occurs with serious sprains. You may hear a crackle or pop with movement. When swelling and pain accompany the sounds and sensations, it's a good bet that some of the ligaments attached to the ankle-joint bones have been hurt.

Another condition is "noisy knees," common when torn knee cartilage sometimes clicks as it catches on the tip of the femur, signaling a possible injury to the meniscus cartilage. Front-of-the-knee pain (patellofemoral pain syndrome) is often accompanied by crunching and crackling, and intensified pain during play and while sitting for long periods with the knee bent.

Noise in itself is not necessarily cause for alarm, unless other symptoms—like tenderness, inflammation, pain, decrease in strength and range of motion, for example—are present.

# The Pelvic Area

There's news both good and bad about the vulnerability of the pelvic area to injury. While serious injuries like fractures are rare, the tendons and muscles in this region are apt to strain. When that occurs, recovery can be slow because this part of the body is never at rest. Pain in the pelvic area can also be difficult to diagnose because it's nonspecific or because it radiates into other parts of the body.

# Injuries to the Coccyx

An awkward fall that lands you flat on your bottom can result in a painful bruise to the coccyx, or tailbone. There's little you can do to speed healing; to

**F.Y.I.**

Key to determining whether or not a groin pain requires prompt medical attention is understanding what caused it. If pain followed a quick twist and turn, it's probably the result of a muscle or tendon strain. If you can't put your finger on a specific triggering incident, consult a physician. Pain in the groin may be due to conditions such as:

• Hernia

• Stress fractures

• Urinary tract infections

• Ovarian cysts

• Testicular tumor

• Arthritis

relieve discomfort, take over-the-counter analgesics and ice the coccyx for about 20 minutes per hour for the first two days. Afterward, apply heat either by using a heating pad or warm towels, or by using a whirlpool. Consult a physician if the pain worsens or you find you can't have a bowel movement.

# Injuries to the Testes

It isn't just football players and other contact-sport athletes who are at risk of taking a hit to the testes. According to Atlanta urologist Steven Morganstern, M.D.: "While football is the number one sport for testicular damage, we also see lots of baseball players, and we see cyclists year round." Softball, basketball, and tennis players are also prone to such injuries.

Surprisingly, among male cyclists, the pressure of sitting on the saddle for long periods of time can injure the testicles and interrupt blood delivery to the groin.

When men get injured in the testes, macho syndrome apparently kicks into full gear. But the decision to tough it out and see a doctor only as a last option can have serious consequences in terms of swelling, decreased blood flow, and, ultimately, tissue damage, tissue death, and sexual dysfunction. When such accidents occur, it's essential to get to a doctor for treatment within six hours.

Pressure or pain in the groin shouldn't be ignored. If a ball socks you in the groin or you begin to suffer cyclist's groin from repetitive pressure, see a physician.

# The Hips

Here's an area that most athletes probably don't give much thought to, and that's certainly because, unlike the arms and legs, the hips aren't the primary body part used in most sports—they don't propel, throw, kick, jump, or swing. They're generally involved in a secondary capacity, facilitating movement for all sports, be it golf, tennis, basketball, swimming, or bowling. Any injury to the hip area can sideline any player for weeks.

## Hip Pointers

If you fall on your side or run into a wall playing racquet sports, you could suffer a hip "pointer"—a painful swelling on the hip caused by a blow to the pelvic area just below the waist. Ice the injury hourly for 20 minutes until the pain abates, returning to play when it's gone.

Athletes at risk for falling or taking a blow on the hips should consider wearing hip football pads to avoid bruising the quads or hips.

## Overuse Injuries of the Hip

Just like other joints in the body, strain and overuse can trigger bursitis of the hip, causing stiffness and pain at the joint, difficulty lying on your side, or difficulty walking or stair climbing. Treat it the way you'd treat inflammation of any other joint—with rest, ice, and aspirin or other anti-inflammatory medicines.

# Injuries to the Hip Adductor Muscles

The quick twists and turns, explosive movements, and cold starts common with recreational activities like racquet sports, skating, and running can literally put a kink in players' pelvic muscles and ligaments. Board certified sports clinical specialist Joe Carroll, M.S., P.T., says that's because "forceful contractions of the large muscles on the inside and front of the thigh can lead to acute groin strains."

What normally happens is that a skater or tennis player competes without properly warming up and then feels something tear. Runners close to finishing a race, athletes who are fatigued, and those who cool down inadequately are apt to injure the hip flexor muscle on the front of the upper thigh or the adductor muscles on the interior of the thigh.

Depending on which muscles or tendons have been strained, you might feel a sudden stabbing pain or tearing sensation in the groin, an inability to pull your leg in toward your body, flex your hips, or rotate your pelvis without considerable pain.

Luckily, acute Grade I injuries can be treated effectively with RICE, with activities back to normal within a few days. To minimize chances of reoccurrence, it's smart to start a series of resistance exercises to strengthen the muscles in the hip, pelvis, and groin once pain has disappeared. A sports trainer or physical therapist can recommend appropriate exercises.

While you can treat a Grade I simple strain yourself, the danger is in ignoring the injury and continuing to play or getting back into sports without addressing one of the underlying problems—

weak muscles in the groin area. If you neglect the initial symptoms and pain progresses to the point that you can't climb stairs without wincing, see a doctor.

# The Thighs and Quads

In fast-paced games like squash, racquetball, tennis, or volleyball, it's easy to take a hit in your quadriceps (muscle on the front of your thigh). A direct blow to the quadriceps—also from falling—can certainly be very painful, leaving behind the imprint of a bad bruise or contusion. If such an injury occurs, ice the muscle with the knee bent. With an ice pack over the muscle, wrap the leg with an elastic bandage so the knee is bent and the calf presses against the hamstrings on the back of the thigh to stop the bleeding into the muscle. Ice the muscle for 20-minute periods as much as possible for the next day.

For injuries that are more than minor, once the icing has been completed, wrap a thick compression pad over the bruise and hold it in place with an elastic bandage. Then it's time to rehab the injured muscles with exercises, like isometric quad sets in which you tighten the thigh muscle and hold for five seconds, repeating 5 to 10 times. If the contusion is really painful, keep the weight off your leg, and use crutches if necessary. Continue the quad rehab exercises and the 20-minute icing sessions (at least three times a day) and start bending your knee as far as possible as long as it doesn't hurt. Use crutches until you can walk painlessly.

Once the pain is under control, it's imperative

## STREET SMARTS

"I've been doing Jazzercise for years, so I was pretty experienced," says Sandra Maple, 48, of San Diego. "In the middle of a recent class, we started to do a twisty step going forward. That's exactly when I felt something pull in my quads. My instructor said it's probably because the muscles on the inside and outside of my thigh aren't as strong as they should be to support the quads. She suggested icing the injury, and modifying steps that required sideways lunges, quick twists, and changes until it healed. That helped, and after about a week, the pain started easing off."

to regain full use of the knee, adding strengthening and conditioning exercises, such as leg raises, stationary biking, and even straight-ahead jogging. Don't rush into squatting, running downhill, and activities that involve quick stops and starts until you've achieved full range of motion and the pain, swelling, and other symptoms have disappeared.

Don't get back into sports without protecting the quads with an impact- or pressure-relief pad like Orthoplast. It is important to protect the quads from reinjury.

Thigh contusions need to be carefully watched because of the possibility of developing a condition called myositis ossificans in which the buildup of scar tissue limits knee flexibility.

# Hamstring Injuries

Little can lay an athlete out faster or with more agony than a pull to the hamstring muscles on the back of the thigh. The primary muscle used in jumping and cycling, athletes at risk for hamstring injuries are those involved in leisure sports requiring quick stops and starts like basketball, cycling, jogging, skiing, skating, volleyball, aerobic dancing, and racquet sports.

As always, inadequate warm-up and stretching are the underpinnings of injury. Add to that poor lower back flexibility and you have an athlete ripe for a hamstring injury. Weak stomach muscles, apparent because the pelvis tilts forward, are also implicated.

Pulls feel like a popped muscle, and are accompanied by acute pain, swelling, and even black and blue bruising on the back of the thigh as blood from the muscle tears seeps downward.

The standard treatment for a hamstring injury is RICE. One or two days later, initiate a program of gentle stretching with the leg raised up on the back of a chair. Grasp your toes, and try to bend your head toward your knee, holding about 10 seconds. Begin with 3 repetitions on each leg, building over time to 10. An alternative exercise is done on your stomach with a light weight attached to the ankle. Slowly stretch the hamstring by lowering it toward the floor and raising it back toward the shoulders. You can get the same effect using hamstring curl equipment at the gym. Perform the same number of reps, building up to 10 as strength and flexibility increase.

# The Knee

This hingelike joint is the largest in the body. It is subject to constant pounding, bending, and twisting from everyday activities, sports, and the impact of falls; as such, injured knees send 6 million people in the United States to the doctor each year.

Depending on the particular condition, the treatments for knee problems range from simply altering lifestyle to total knee replacement.

## Injuries to the Anterior Cruciate Ligament (ACL)

The last thing an athlete wants to incur is an injury to the anterior cruciate ligament (ACL). As one of seven ligaments connecting the bones at the knee joint, it's essential to stabilizing the knee. Unfortu-

### STREET SMARTS

Real estate investor Denis Cramer, 51, reckons he's done 10,000 running miles. "Just like a car's tires, my kneecap became misaligned as a result of all that shock and wear and tear," he says. "The pain got so bad that I had to quit running, playing golf, and couldn't even manage a flight of stairs." The problem for Cramer was multifold: his quadriceps (responsible for helping to support the kneecap) were weak, so the kneecap moved off center. This caused the patellar (kneecap) to rub against the femur, wearing down connective cartilage. "The solution was to strengthen the quads with physical therapy," he says. "Within a few months, I was back in the game!"

nately for athletes who play sports like tennis or basketball, which involve rapid running with quick changes of direction or drops in speed, the odds of sustaining an injury to the ACL are higher than for any other part of the knee. Located in the middle of the knee, it crosses the posterior cruciate ligament (PCL) to help keep the thigh and shin bones from sliding out of position. An athlete who hears a pop, feels the knee "give," followed by pain and swelling has most likely strained or ruptured the ligament. According to the National Hospital Discharge Survey, in 1994 there were 50,000 hospital admissions for repair of the ACL and posterior cruciate ligaments in the knee.

Like sprains elsewhere in the body, ACL injuries are graded in seriousness from first to third degree, with first degree being the most mild. While these usually heal with one or two weeks of rest, third-degree ruptures used to be considered career-ending injuries until techniques to transplant the ACL tendon from a cadaver or an allograft (from one's own body) of a patellar tendon and bone were developed.

# Kneecap Pain (Patellofemoral Pain)

Characterized by pain in front of or around the kneecap when bending, going downstairs, running downhill, or after prolonged sitting, the problem is often caused by imbalances in muscle strength. While the outer quads in the thighs are tight and strong, the muscles of the inner thigh are not, so the kneecap is pulled off balance. Anatomical discrepancies in leg length, flat feet, and inward turn-

# Treating Injuries Naturally

Not every athlete wants to pop a Tylenol or a prescription drug to treat pains, strains, and inflammations, especially when the same or similar effect might be had from herbs and vitamins. Here are some to check out:

- **Turmeric.** Touted as a natural anti-inflammatory agent, turmeric contains an active ingredient, curcumin, claimed to relieve redness, swelling, and pain when the spice is rubbed directly into a sprain. One reason for its effectiveness is that it contains vitamin C, crucial for tissue repair, and has an antihistamine effect on inflammation, reducing swelling. In addition to eating the vividly colored yellow-orange spice in Indian food, you can get it in various other forms from a holistic or Oriental medicine practitioner.

- **Ginger.** According to two small 1989 Danish studies by researchers at Odense University, ginger rivals nonsteroidal anti-inflammatory drugs in terms of reducing swelling and relieving pain. The Herb Research Foundation says that ginger is used to effect pain relief in dosages of 400 to 500 milligrams four times daily. Though the foundation refers to some experts that "caution against the use of ginger during pregnancy," it concludes that "there is little evidence of any significant risk from ginger when used at moderate doses."

- **Echinacea.** In addition to its positive affect on the immune system, echinacea has been found to aid wound healing and reduce inflammation, says Daniel Mowrey, Ph.D., author of *Herbal Tonic Therapies* and *The Scientific Validation of Herbal Medicine*.

- **Vitamin E.** A study by William J. Evans, Ph.D., professor of applied physiology and director of the Noll Physiological Research Center at Pennsylvania State University reported that vitamin E may have surprising healing applications for weekend exercisers. He found that vitamin E quickens healing of the microscopic tears in muscles that develop as a result of vigorous exercise, and reduces the production of oxygen-free radicals. The study, which focused on older, active people, found that vitamin E supplements would not be necessary for endurance athletes, whose metabolisms already work efficiently.

## SMART MOVE

"Target training the quad, abs, and calf is the best way to prevent skiing injuries," says Catherine S. Hoell, M.S., P.T., in *Training Tips for Knee-Friendly Skiing,* published online by Cape Cod Rehabilitation. "Most injuries occur not by underdeveloped quadricep muscles, but by muscle imbalances. For example, you may spend your preseason workouts doing crunches, leg extensions, and calf raises, but these exercises must be balanced with exercises for shin, hamstring, and back extensor muscles. Otherwise, your quads have to work in overdrive to compensate for weak hamstrings. It's when muscles get tired that falls are most likely to occur. Also, when muscles are in balance, you use less energy to ski."

ing thighbones also put the athlete at risk for kneecap pain. Sports that put athletes at risk for this injury are those which involve considerable running like racquet sports and basketball.

If the condition is caused by muscle weakness, strengthening exercises will set things right. Anatomical abnormalities may require the wearing of a knee brace or other orthotic.

Here are some suggestions from the *Healthwise Handbook* to prevent knee problems from developing:

• Eliminate knee bends or squats from exercise.

• Skip downhill runs unless you're in top form.

• Choose athletic shoes that have excellent arch supports, and replace running shoes after three hundred miles.

## Jumper's Knee

Volleyball and basketball players are prone to inflammation of the tendons that attach to the top and bottom of the kneecap. Responsible for helping the leg to straighten, the quadriceps and patellar tendons are apt to become inflamed with repetitive upright jumping. Jumper's knee can be slow to heal because of limited blood supply to the tendons. But if the condition is mild with pain present only during or immediately after play, it might be treated successfully with RICE followed by moist heat 72 hours later.

The biggest challenge to the athlete with jumper's knee is to develop patience. If you return to play too soon, the whole cycle will start again, and may lead eventually to surgery. That may mean staying away from the sport that precipitated the problem for as long as a month.

## Meniscus Cartilage Tears

The same old culprits that cause a plethora of sports injuries—quick twists, violent muscle contractions, overuse of an injured knee, or a blow to the knee—are behind yet another sports malady, meniscus cartilage tears. Characterized by swelling and pain upon injury, followed by stiffness and inability to straighten or bend the knee, cartilage or ligament tears can make the knee joint feel wobbly. The injury is deceptive because while the knee begins to feel better after RICE, you're often pretty much back to pain once you start sports again.

**SMART DEFINITION**

**Meniscus injury**

This is a damage to cartilage (bone) in the knee at the top of the lower leg bone (tibia).

## Moves to Prevent Knee Injuries While Skiing

The chain of events precipitating a skiing accident are often subtle and happen so quickly that a skier who hasn't mentally prepared for such possibilities can get seriously injured. Here are some suggestions to make falls easier by decreasing the stress of twisting on the knee as the desperate skier flails about attempting to keep upright:

• If you feel as if you're falling, bring your arms forward.

• Move your feet closer together and make sure your knees remain in line and under your hips.

• Position your hands over the skis.

*Source: Training Tips for Knee-Friendly Skiing,* published online by Cape Cod Rehabilitation

"Being the manager of a gym, I obviously should have known better," says Peter Dufour, 34, manager of Fitness West in San Diego. "I'd just gone down to the rec center and a group of guys were looking for someone for a pick-up game of basketball, so I jumped in. I was dribbling down the forecourt, twisting and turning the way you do, and I felt something go in my knee. I got the knee rehabed, but once you injure that part of the body, it's always going to be the weak link in the anatomical chain. Eventually one injury led to another and I had to have arthroscopic surgery. All this because I didn't take the time to warm up and stretch."

This is one injury that almost certainly will require surgery to remove the damaged cartilage because there just isn't enough blood supply to the bone to promote recovery. Fortunately, the days of operations requiring a large incision on the knee, several days of hospitalization with considerable pain and extensive rehabilitation are over. Today, the torn part of the cartilage can be removed arthroscopically with a fiber-optic instrument that has a lighted tip. The procedure involves very small incisions and often same day surgery, followed with physical therapy and rehab exercises.

Small cartilage tears and those at the outer edge of the cartilage are possible exceptions to surgery. Under intense rehabilitation, this may heal so that the athlete is back in the game within about a month.

With so much at risk, it makes sense to prevent cartilage tears whenever possible. As always, this means being sure to strengthen and condition the knee before you undertake vigorous play, warm up sufficiently so the joint can move easily, and avoid running or playing on concrete or asphalt surfaces. If you've had a previous knee injury, protect it from further damage by taping it.

# Safe Guidelines for Knee Rehabilitation

Once you've injured your knee, the road back to full sports participation involves rehabilitation exercises to strengthen the muscles in your legs. Whether you choose to join a gym or fitness center for access to exercise equipment after suffering a knee injury is a matter of personal choice. But whatever your decision, follow these sensible guidelines from *At-Home Knee Rehabilitation: Stengthening Wihout Special Equipment* by Kris Jensen, M.S., P.T., S.C.S.:

• Don't assume that there's a one-size-fits-all rehab program for knee injuries. Follow your doctor's or physical therapist's recommendations and discontinue any exercises that cause significant pain during or after the session.

• Your leg muscles need time to recoup, so don't push yourself. Perform your rehab exercises every other day.

• The number of reps of each exercise you do will depend on your overall condition, the number of exercises, and what you hope to achieve in the initial session. Start conservatively with one set of 6 to 12 reps for each exercise. As you become stronger, gradually increase to four sets of 6 to 12 repetitions with one- to two-minute rests in between. Increase the difficulty of exercises by upping the reps or shortening the rest periods.

## Ensuring Knee Function

Once a knee injury has healed and range of motion has been restored through rehabilitation exercises, an athlete still isn't ready to get back in the game. The final link in the healing chain is "functional progression, an orderly sequence of activities enabling the athlete to reacquire the physical tools necessary for a safe return to the court," reports the *Penn State Sports Medicine Newsletter.*

John Darmelio, A.T.C., of the Methodist Sports

When you hurt yourself playing sports, it's tempting to reach for nonsteroidal anti-inflammatory drugs (NSAIDs) immediately. But that could be a big mistake. A report in the *Sports Science Exchange* warned that NSAID usage shouldn't begin until 72 hours after the injury. "If used too early, NSAIDs may block the collection of platelets and add to the initial swelling," says the report. "Their use 72 hours or more after the injury can reduce pain and provide much-needed anti-inflammatory benefits."

Medicine Clinic of Indianapolis, Indiana, has developed a prototype of a functional progression program adaptable to basketball, volleyball, and other court sports. The key to the program is to stay tuned to your body, only going on to the next step once the previous one has been accomplished without pain or limping. Once you've completed the program, you can go back to playing, though it may be advisable to wear a knee brace.

# The Calf and Shin

The calf (the large muscle in the back of the leg below the knee) and the shin (the front part of the lower leg from the knee to the ankle) are also subject to stress, injury, and damage from sports activities, misuse, and poor conditioning.

## Shinsplints

If you run, aerobic dance, play volleyball or similar running sports, you've probably seen how repetitive pounding of the feet can lead to tenderness, pain, or swelling on the back or inside part of the shin (lower leg). What's actually happened is that doing too much exercise without appropriate rest or suddenly increasing the amount of exercise has caused an overuse injury affecting the muscles near the shin bone. You may notice that the pain is worse when you start playing, decreases as you continue, and is at its worst when the game is over or after you wake up the next day.

Shinsplints located in the front of the shin bone (tibia) are called anterior shinsplints.

Shinsplints on the inside of the leg along the tibia bone are called posterior shinsplints. Both result from minute muscle tears in the area that attaches to the shin bone.

According to the American Running and Fitness Association, "tight calf muscles on the back and side of the calf, which propel the body forward, place additional strain on the muscles in the front part of the lower leg, which lift the foot upward, preparing it to strike the running surface."

The type of shoes an athlete wears or the surfaces on which he runs or plays also can cause shinsplints. When shoes become worn, losing their ability to absorb shock, or exercise is performed on hard surfaces, muscles on the front of the leg are stressed, causing anterior shinsplints.

Runners whose gait is off because contact with the ground is made only with the balls of their feet rather than with their heels (called toe running) are at risk for anterior shinsplints.

So too are those whose feet tend to overpronate, turning in during running. "This forces the muscles of the foot and leg to overwork in an attempt to stabilize the foot, resulting in muscle tears," the association points out.

To both treat and prevent shinsplints, remember to gently stretch the muscles in the back of the legs and the thigh muscles before and after playing. Icing the area after playing, treating the inflammation and pain with aspirin or ibuprofen, cutting back on how much running you do, and switching to more forgiving surfaces for running, tennis, and aerobic dancing will relieve the symptoms.

Athletes prone to shinsplints should forego running on hills. For those whose problems are caused by feet that turn in, the association suggests adding a varus wedge to their shoes in order to support the inside of the foot, thereby reducing the amount of pronation. As always, athletes who put the time in to strengthen and condition their bodies to correct muscle imbalances will help prevent shinsplints from occurring and will heal more quickly should injuries strike.

## Strengthening Exercises to Prevent Shinsplints

To prevent shinsplints, try these exercises recommended by Brian Metiner, ATC, published by UW Health University Physician and Physicians Plus:

• **Runner's stretch:** With hands shoulder distance apart, place hands on the wall as if performing upright push-ups. With your left leg extended back and your right knee bent, stretch the left leg by bringing your heel to the ground. Hold at least 20 seconds. Alternate legs, doing three to five reps on each leg prior to and after playing. When the back of the calves are flexible, the front of the legs are less likely to be stressed and incur shinsplints.

• **Leg and calf raises:** Seated on a chair, raise both legs so they're fully extended, but don't lock the knees. Alternate with one-leg calf raises. Hold each for about three seconds to strengthen the posterior calf muscles.

• **Heel walking:** Leaning back on your heels with toes raised off the ground, flex your ankle, strengthening the front of the calf.

• **Pick-up toes:** Strengthen your arches by using your toes to pick up tissues from the floor.

## Achilles Tendinitis

The largest of the body's tendons, the Achilles connects calf muscles to the heel. Athletes who do sports involving lots of jumping, like basketball or aerobic dancing, as well as those whose feet roll in when they walk or run can wind up with an inflammation of the Achilles tendon. Symptoms of pain and swelling are easily treated with anti-inflammatory medications, icing, and stretches to increase tendon flexibility, such as the runner's stretch.

# The Ankle and Heel

The quick twists and turns inherent in playing many sports make the ankle joint one of the most often injured in athletics. Because injuries here are so frequent, there has been considerable research on how to treat hurt ankles for the quickest recovery.

The heel is subject to constant pounding daily, even when not playing sports. The most common heel injury, however, can be avoided.

## Ankle Sprains

Ankle sprains, the most common reason for emergency room visits, account for almost one out of every five sports-related injuries. More than 27,000 ankle sprains occur daily in the United States. And 45 percent of basketball injuries and 24 percent of volleyball injuries are ankle sprains.

The usual scenario for an ankle sprain is an un-

**F.Y.I.**

If your ankle tends to twist when you do sports involving walking, running, or jumping, help may be just a shoe away. Here are suggestions from the American Orthopaedic Foot and Ankle Society:

• Switch to shoes with a firm heel counter.

• Runners with weak ankles should try shoes that also have a moderately flared heel.

• Racquet-sports players need shoes that have a high cut.

• Alpine ski boots provide good ankle support for skiers.

• Wearing a brace to keep the ankle stable also helps.

expected turning in of the ankle so that the sole winds up exposed and facing the opposite foot. This contortion stresses the ankle's outside ligaments, resulting in a sudden pain, a popping sensation, and swelling.

Generally considered a minor injury, ankle sprains often can be treated with RICE immediately after the injury followed by a short period of immobilization and protection with bandaging, taping, or bracing to control pain and swelling. More severe sprains may require a cast, brace, and in rare instances, surgery.

Like other sprains, its severity is reflected in whether it's graded as a I, II, or III injury. The AOFAS says that "most ankle sprains are mild, involving stretched ligaments with no tear (Grade I injury)." When the extent of the injury can be established by physical examination alone and X-rays aren't needed, the ankle is protected with adhesive strapping so that the athlete can continue cycling, swimming, even running. The key to recuperating is to avoid situations in which the ankle is forced to twist, at least for the next couple of weeks.

To determine if a tear has actually occurred, dye is injected into the the joint or tendon in a procedure called an arthrogram or tenogram.

A Grade II injury involving a partial ligament tear will require a cast for two to four weeks. Athletes may continue working out, says the AOFAS, if they wear a fiberglass cast.

No such luck if you incur a Grade III complete ligament tear. Medical opinion on this type of injury is split between those who believe that surgery is required and others who advocate allowing the injury to heel on its own immobilized in a plaster cast for six weeks. Still others say that thanks to new braces, wraps, and aggressive rehabiliation, athletes can return to normal in just a week or so. Which is best? According to the AOFAS, new research shows that putting the ankle in a brace early in the injury and keeping it there for six weeks results in as good or better recovery than immobilization and surgical repair. Most patients in the study returned to work in one to seven weeks and were back into sports within seven weeks to three months.

Once in a while, an athlete will experience several episodes of twisting the ankle. That could result in surgery to build a new ankle ligament via grafting healthy tissue from other nearby tendons. Other surgeons prefer to repair the damage without grafts by using small incisions to shorten the stretched ligament back into shape. Such reconstructive surgery, followed by a walking cast for up to a month, has about an 85 percent success rate, according to the AOFAS. To complete the healing process, exercises to strengthen the ankle are required.

# Prompt Treatment Prevents Disability

Getting prompt medical treatment for sprains involving the midfoot can prevent prolonged disability and chronic pain. That's the case when athletes land on the ball of the foot and it rotates out, injuring the tarsometatarsal joint near where the toes meet the arch. According to a study at the Union Memorial Hospital in Baltimore, athletes who injure this joint and don't seek prompt care still suffer pain and inability to play sports two years later.

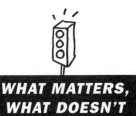

**WHAT MATTERS, WHAT DOESN'T**

*Treating a Sprained Ankle*

## What Matters

• Knowing if the ankle can bear weight; if it can't, it's more seriously injured.

• Not sabotaging the healing process by returning to play too quickly. Sprains can take six to eight weeks to heal.

• Getting medical attention within 24 to 48 hours if pain and swelling interfere with standing or walking.

## What Doesn't

• Having every ankle sprain X-rayed. X-rays are indicated only when there's pain directly over the ankle bone or the back edge of the ankle, when the ankle can't bear weight, or if you're over 55.

• Extent of bruising. Even minor sprains cause discoloration, so the bruise tells little.

**F.Y.I.**

• A decade long study measuring patient satisfaction in terms of conservative treatment for plantar fasciitis reveals that casting the injury was most effective.

• The second most effective treatment was steroid injections, according to patients.

• Of the approximately four hundred patients in the study, 61 percent were female, and half stood on their feet for long hours. More than 75 percent were overweight, considered a significant contributor factor in developing the condition.

Unlike most ankle sprains that generally get better on their own without treatment, about 75 percent with this type of injury suffer long-lasting problems.

Such injuries are difficult to diagnose, notes the AOFAS, because injuries may not show up on an X-ray. The only way to get an accurate read on what's happened to the foot is to examine it under local anesthesia. If the joint is sprained, the injury may be treated either with a nonweight bearing plaster cast or surgery.

# Plantar Fasciitis and Heel Spurs

When you get a sharp pain inside your heel or arch with the first few steps getting out of bed, you probably have plantar fasciitis. What's deceptive about this condition is that it seems to disappear as you play, only to resurface with a vengence if you jump at the end of a workout.

The most prevalent cause of heel pain, inflammation of the plantar fascia, the fibrous tissue running from base of the toes to the heel, is the result of tiny tears near the heel. The culprits are overuse, running on surfaces with too much or too little give, and errors in training, such as inadequate rest between workouts. Of course, those who have insufficient ankle and foot strength or flexibility, flat feet, and high arches are also at risk because feet that roll over add additional strain to the heel.

If left untreated, the heel can grow additional bone, forming a heel spur.

## Shoe Design Can Reduce Injury Risk

One of the easiest ways to prevent a variety of foot problems affecting the heel and shin is to buy shoes properly designed to compensate for common foot conditions. Here are some recommendations from the American Orthopaedic Foot and Ankle Society (AOFAS):

• **Plantar Fascia.** What's needed here is superb shock absorption in the heel. Adding a heel pad or wedge can also minimize stress on the midheel. If you already have plantar fasciitis, the AOFAS recommends "foam pads with a cut-out or orthotics with a well-cushioned heel and a well to float the painful area. A shoe with a firm medial heel counter can decrease tendency for the foot to turn in and stress on the plantar fascia."

• **Bursitis.** Poorly fitting shoes and insufficient padding in the heel counter can cause the bursa surrounding the Achilles tendon to become inflamed. The remedy is to get a new pair of athletic shoes "with well-padded heel counter, an Achilles notch (a depression in the back of the counter to relieve pressure on the tendon), and a heel height of at least 15 millimeters."

• **Achilles Tendon.** Surprisingly, shoes with a relatively low heel can be partially to blame for Achilles tendinitis. But the condition can be avoided with shoes that have a well padded-tendon pad or notch, and the addition of heel lifts to raise the foot in the shoe, relieving tendon tension. The AOFAS also says that shoes with "a firm heel counter can reduce the side-to-side motion of the heel and tendon, thus reducing irritation of the tendon."

# The Toes

What sports injuries can do to your toes makes you want to bury them in sand. Breaks, dislocations, bruises, neuromas—it's a lot for tiny digits to take. But here are some tips to help keep toes in tiptop shape.

# Shoe Lacing to Prevent Injuries and Pain

The way in which you lace your athletic shoes can actually prevent injuries and alleviate pain and a host of foot problems. Here are some tips on changing the lacing patterns on shoes with double rows of eyelets to address specific foot concerns:

• **Narrow Feet:** If you have narrow feet, consider using the eyelets set wider on the shoe (see figure A). This will bring up the sides of the shoe more tightly across the top of the narrow foot.

• **Wide Feet:** If you have wide feet, consider using the eyelets closer to the tongue of the shoe (see figure B). Using the eyelets that are closer together will give more width to the lacing area and have the same effect as letting out a corset.

• **Narrow Heel and Wide Forefoot:** If you have a narrow heel and a wide ball of the foot or forefoot, consider using two laces to achieve a combination fit (see figure C). Use both sets of eyelets to achieve a custom fit that accommodates the width of the forefoot and tightens around the narrow heel. Use the closer-set eyelets to adjust the width of the shoe at the forefoot and the wide-set eyelets to snug up the heel.

• **Specific Pain:** If you have a bump on the top of your foot, a high arch, a bone that sticks out, or pain from a nerve or tendon injury, consider leaving a space in the lacing to alleviate pressure (see figure D). Simply skip the eyelets at the point of pain and draw the laces to the next set of eyelets. This lacing pattern will greatly increase the comfort of the shoe.

• **High Arches:** If you have a high arch, consider lacing your shoes so that the laces travel in a straight line from eyelet to eyelet (see figure E). By avoiding the criss-cross method, this lacing pattern creates no pressure points at the laces.

• **Toe Problems:** Hammer toes, corns, bleeding toes, or nail problems? Lacing your shoe so the toe-box area is lifted can help considerably (see figure F). You can adjust the height of the toe box by pulling on the lace that travels directly from the toe to the top of the shoe.

• **Heel Fit:** To prevent heel blisters, try the lacing pattern in figure G. Notice that the top laces are threaded through each other before tying the shoe.

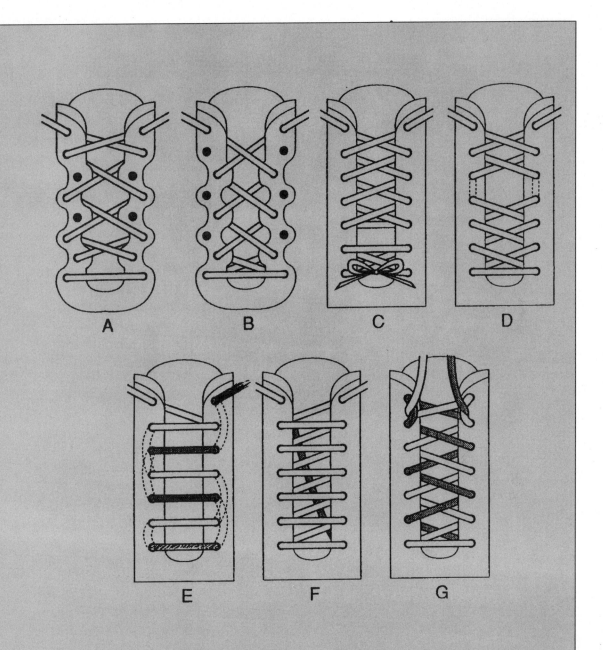

*Source:* Carol Frey, M.D., chief, Foot and Ankle Clinic at the University of Southern California and the American Orthopaedic Foot and Ankle Society

# In-Grown and Discolored Toenails

The discomfort of in-grown toenails and the un-sightliness of black toenails, though no major ath-letic crisis, are still concerns to be addressed. The solution to these may be as near as your neighbor-hood sports-supply store.

The prevailing causes of these conditions are tight-fitting shoes or shoes that are simply too small, so that the big toe slams against the end of the toe box. This makes the toe bleed under the toenail, which then turns black, eventually falling off. Changing to an athletic shoe with a comfort-ably wide and high toe box should solve this un-sightly problem.

In-grown toenails can be caused by faulty nail care—cutting the nails in such a way that jagged edges cut into skin of other toes.

# Corns

These result from pressure on the toes from the toe box. If the athlete has hammer toes that bend up at the middle joint, wearing shoes that don't fit properly because they are too short or narrow can cause a corn to develop on the joint. To eliminate this problem, use doughnut-shaped pads or lamb's wool over the toe, and change to a high toe box and a better-fitting shoe.

# Broken Toes

If something falls on your toe or you slam it, the pain can be excruciating, making it difficult to tell a strain from a break. An X-ray will not only determine if it's actually broken but at what angle the fracture has occurred so that the doctor knows to which neighbor the injured one should be bound. Without an X-ray, the injury could be taped to the wrong toe, making the fracture, like a crack, pull wider apart.

To make walking less painful, use a shoe with a stiff sole to minimize toe movement when walking. If you break your toe, healing is made easy by binding it to a neighboring toe with tape.

# Interdigital Neuroma

Wearing shoes that are too narrow or performing sports like aerobic dancing in which there's excessive pressure on the ball of the foot can cause an interdigital neuroma, a pinched nerve in the webspace between the middle and fourth toes. Usually, the pain will disappear if you give the foot a rest from the sport causing the problem, along with ice massage and aspirin, ibuprofen, or acetaminophen. To prevent reoccurrence, you'll need new, wider shoes with shock absorption that extends into the forefooot. Ask the salesman to show you shoes with various types of rocker soles specifically adapted to decrease heel strike and relieve pressure on the foot. Try a foam pad from the drugstore to place under the ball of your foot to relieve pressure. Your physician can also prescribe orthotics to relieve pressure on the nerve.

**SMART DEFINITION**

**Heel counter**

The heel counter is the rear part of the shoe that cups the heel.

**Achilles notch**

The Achilles notch is a depression in the back of the counter and is designed to relieve pressure on the Achilles tendon.

**Rocker sole**

A rocker sole has been modified at various positions to relieve or transfer pressure from designated areas of the foot and ankle.

## THE BOTTOM LINE

Shoes are the culprits of many athletic injuries. Footwear that's too narrow or short can cause a variety of injuries to the toes and foot, which can be relieved just by having new shoes properly fitted for your feet. Lacing is also important in foot care. Depending on the anatomy of your foot, changing the way in which you lace your shoes can go a long way to preventing injuries and relieving pain.

When we're hurt, it's easy to overreact because of the way the injury looks. A badly bruised foot might send us in search of immediate medical care. But it need not. Just because the ankle or foot is badly discolored doesn't necessarily indicate it's sprained or even broken.

For men, injuries to the testes can result in serious problems if not promptly treated.

If pain persists and the problem is obviously related to your foot's anatomy—large, bony bumps on your toe joints, for example—the problem may require surgery.

# Nerve Entrapment

Poorly fitting shoes are the culprit here as well, since irritating footwear like ski boots and ice skates can put pressure on nerves near the skin's surface. Shoes that are padded and fit correctly will alleviate the pain. A change in the lacing technique will also relieve pressure.

An athlete in motion is a thing of power, grace, and beauty. How quickly you move in on a shot, the ease with which you jump to return a volleyball serve, or the surefootedness with which you rotate on your feet to perform the intricacies of an aerobic dance depend on the condition of your pelvis and lower extremities. With careful attention to warming up and conditioning, you up chances of enjoying leisure sports without time off for inury.

# Preventing and Treating Injuries:

## Sport by Sport

## THE KEYS

• Wearing sport-specific shoes that have been properly fitted can prevent many injuries.

• Orthotics can correct biomechanical problems that predispose athletes to injury.

• Sport "unfriendly" surfaces like concrete and hills can increase injury rate.

• To prevent becoming hurt when using a different court or playing field, get a feel for the new surface before getting into the game.

In any sport, preventing injury is the most essential part of your training regimen. "Studies show most injuries occur during training," says Donald Baxter, M.D., AOFAS president and team physician for several Olympic runners. "When injuries such as pulled hamstrings or Achilles tendonosis or tendinitis occur, it is difficult for an athlete to perform at his or her peak."

Here are sport-by-sport specifics on the most common injuries and how to prevent them, along with some recommendations on treatment if you happen to become one of the unfortunates. (For more detailed information on the prevention and treatment of many of the injuries covered here, refer to chapters 3, 4, 5, and 8.)

# Running

## Common Injuries

• Stress fractures

• Blisters

• Black toenails

• Achilles tendon injuries

• Peritendinitis

• Heel pain

Running injuries normally have an easily discernible cause and effect. If you begin developing pain with running, Baxter suggests you ask yourself these questions:

• Have I recently increased my training mileage?

• Have I made any recent change in shoewear? Did I rotate my shoes among two or three types to avoid similar stresses? Did I notice a specific abnormal wear pattern?

• What type of surface do I run on? Is it hard or soft, circular or slanted?

• Do I maintain a routine of stretching or yoga? Do I use weights to build up strength in a balanced manner?

• Do I drink sufficient amounts of water with training, racing, and hot weather conditions?

Get problems resolved early on; even minor ones like black toenails and blisters can ruin the activity. Prevent foot blisters by wearing a metatarsal pad to take pressure off blister-prone areas.

## Stress Fractures

According to the American Orthopaedic Foot and Ankle Society (AOFAS), the most common cause of stress fracture is an increase in the amount or intensity of exercise resulting in fatigued muscles. This can lead to decreased shock absorption, which places high loads on bones. Running on hard surfaces, wearing an improper supportive shoe, or sustaining an injury to an opposite extremity can lead to a stress fracture.

In a stress fracture, the bone is cracked only

partially. It remains stable and usually can continue bearing weight safely. The runner who develops a stress fracture may experience a vague aching in the affected area for weeks or months. This may suddenly become more painful, forcing him to visit a physician.

Treatment for the majority of stress fractures consists of discontinuing or reducing the amount of running. Athletes can take up swimming, biking, rowing, or weight training instead. If the injury occurs in the foot, an orthosis (orthopaedic insert) will help to relieve symptoms. A cast rarely is necessary.

## Achilles Tendon Injuries

Although an Achilles tendon rupture isn't common, chronic Achilles tendinitis is. Stretching the calf muscles can help (the muscles of the calf come together to form the Achilles tendon, which attaches to the back of the heel). However, according to the AOFAS, Achilles tendon injuries may be difficult to treat and can become chronic.

Runners who run on the forefoot develop a peritendinitis (involving the tendon sheath rather than the tendon itself) directly behind the prominence on the back of the ankle (malleolus). Stop running for several weeks, apply RICE, take an anti-inflammatory medication, use heel lifts, and even try a new pair of shoes. Persistent problems may require a month's stint in a short-leg walking cast designed to preclude running and to heal the tendon. Occasionally surgery is needed if all conservative treatment fails.

## Heel Pain

Heel pain is the most common foot problem among runners. Most runners who complain of heel pain have plantar fasciitis, or pain at the attachment of the plantar fascia (the strong tissue that stretches from the heel to the ball of the foot). Treat with RICE, anti-inflammatory medications, and arch supports (often worn for several months). As a result of the inflammation, and because of the tension produced by the fascia, a bony spur may gradually form on the heel. Some runners may irritate a nerve near the heel and may need surgery to decompress the nerve.

Initially, the symptoms appear gradually, and the athlete carries on with training. The symptoms often will worsen, and the plantar fascia can actually rupture away from the heel, causing a sharp, knifelike pain and a possible disability for 6 to 12 weeks.

The AOFAS recommends treatment that includes rest, a heel cup, a soft heel pad or flexible orthosis with a heel wedge, plus stretching four times a day for 20 seconds. Other treatments include ice, ultrasound treatment, or occasionally corticosteroid injections. When the athlete is pain free on rising in the morning, she can begin a graduated running program.

## Biomechanical Problems

Athletes sometimes have biomechanical problems that can lead to injury. Biomechanical problems occur when an athlete doesn't use a body part in the correct or most efficient manner to perform a task, such as throwing a ball or lifting something heavy. A common biomechanical problem is over-pronation. Runners often talk about pronation, or

**SMART DEFINITION**

**Pronation**

Pronation is an excessive rolling-in of the foot when walking.

**Supination**

Supination is an excessive rolling-out of the foot when walking.

**Orthoses**

Orthoses are custom shoe inserts that can be prescribed by a podiatrist or other physician.

turning out of the hindfoot (the position that the foot tries to assume if you exaggerate a knock-kneed appearance). Some pronation is normal and necessary for fluid running, to help absorb shock. Excessive pronation may lead to arch fatigue and knee pain or even dislocation of the kneecap. Placing an arch support and occasionally a heel wedge in the running shoe may diminish pronation of the foot and correct the knee pain. Some running shoes already have built-in heel wedges.

Many inexpensive, over-the-counter orthotics are readily available in different sizes. With the improved quality of construction in running shoes and the substantial arch supports provided in many shoes, most people no longer need an expensive, custom-molded orthosis.

## Short-Leg Syndrome

A short leg may be the result of a congenital problem or from running on the same tilt of the road or the same direction on a circular track. Runners with a leg length inequality often suffer stress fractures, knee strain, plantar fasciitis, knee-cap dislocation, and tendinitis to the short leg. Athletes also can develop a quadriceps strain from weakness of the shorter leg. A physician can correct a short leg by adding a lift to the inner lining of the shoe. Occasionally problems such as hip pain develop in the long leg.

## Malalignment Problems

Runners with a high arch or pronated feet are susceptible to overuse injuries affecting the back and knee. Being bowlegged, knock-kneed, or toeing in or out also lead to problems secondary to the stress of running.

If your feet do pronate, an over-the-counter soft orthosis may correct the problem. Some runners may need semiflexible orthotic constructed of heat-sensitive materials. Occasionally a rigid orthosis may be recommended, although the AOFAS suggests these be avoided since they can lead to stress fractures. Orthoses that must be individually made require the skills of someone who understands the biomechanics of the foot.

## Preventing Runner's Injuries

To help reduce chances of becoming injured:

• Stay a step ahead of sports-related injuries by wearing the right shoes with the right fit.

• Avoid prolonged running on slanted surfaces.

• Avoid sprinting or sudden bursts of speed that can cause violent jolts and ruptures of tendons and muscles.

• Take one or two days off per week to recuperate.

• Try to run on grass or dirt rather than concrete.

## Treating Running Injuries

If you develop running injuries, here are some general guidelines from the AOFAS that may be helpful:

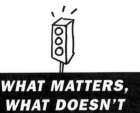

### WHAT MATTERS, WHAT DOESN'T

**What Matters**

• Not running a major race in new shoes.

• Making sure laces are tightly tied.

• Starting with a slow walk progressing to a slow jog before picking up speed.

• Warming up and stretching before participating in any sport.

• Taking days off between training.

**What Doesn't**

• Training daily to try to maintain a competitive edge.

• Buying the latest name brand running shoes.

• Change training to run within the limits of pain.

• Alter stride length and pace to eliminate symptoms.

• Change to a soft, less-slanted surface with minimal curves that allows sliding such as grass or cinders.

• Stretch. Yoga helps with stretching in a rotational direction. Strengthening exercises with weights can help some athletes. Numerous repetitions with light weights increase muscle endurance.

• Apply ice to the area after swelling. Heat will often benefit if there is minimal swelling and when there are body areas that need increased circulation.

• Try low-impact exercises such as bicycle riding or swimming.

• Take aspirin three to four times a day for one to two weeks. Take aspirin only during periods of reduced running to avoid dehydration and other fluid problems.

• Surgery should be consider only as a last resort. Investigate thsi option fully only only after 6 to 12 months of conservative treatment.

# Previous Injuries Influence Performance

When performance fails to live up to expectations, the reason may be as simple as a sprained ankle sustained in the previous year.

Inadequate rehabilitation of previous injuries is a major contributor to existing and future problems. The absence of symptoms doesn't mean the athlete has fully recovered or is ready to perform at peak level. Even an injury as deceptively simple as a sprained ankle can lead to serious performance problems if only the symptoms are treated. Swelling and pain may disappear, but if the loss of balance associated with an ankle sprain is not addressed, there is a great chance of a recurrent sprain within six months.

What's needed is a comprehensive rehabilitative approach. "Not only do we need to make a complete and accurate diagnosis of the problem, but also we need to treat alterations in flexibility, strength, balance, and gait caused by the injury," says Stan Herring, M.D., rehabilitation doctor and physician for the Seattle Seahawks football team. "We need to identify the tissues overloaded and any functional changes present. Athletes also have a tendency to adapt their sports style because of pain or discomfort, and this needs to be addressed as well."

The final part of the rehabilitation equation is the ability to demonstrate sport-specific skills. For example, a football player who can't do lateral drills or a basketball player who can't perform stopping and starting drills shouldn't return to the sport.

"Athletes have to meet several goals for a re-

## SMART MOVE

"Previous injury is a major factor in poor performance problems," says Stan Herring, M.D., rehabilitation doctor and physician for the Seattle Seahawks football team. "Previous injury also is the best predictor of future injury, particularly among those who return to activity too soon. Those who return to sports early get injured very rapidly once they are back in the game."

turn to sports, including a full range of motion, symmetrical strength, endurance, power, good flexibility, and demonstrated sport-specific skills," says Herring. "Only when these goals are met is the athlete ready to return to sports and perform at a high level."

# Running in Winter

Runners are more prone to injury in cold weather from failure to warm up sufficiently, leaving the body at risk for pulls, tears, and strains.

Whether consciously or unconsciously, runners may change their foot-strike pattern to protect themselves, leading to muscle strain or overuse injuries. To increase traction, runners may land on slippery surfaces with the whole foot instead of the natural rolling action of the heel-to-toe strike. Lateral slippage could result in a painful groin pull.

If a runner must jog on ice, spikes slipped over running shoes may be helpful, but only if you've practiced with them on other surfaces like a running track. Strangely enough, even moving feet can suffer frostbite because cold can penetrate the thin material of running shoes. Tight shoes increase chances of frostbite.

# Aerobic Dancing

## Common Injuries

- Plantar fasciitis

- Heel spurs

- Sesamoiditis

- Shin splints

- Achilles tendon and calf pain

- Stress fractures

- Low back pain

Aerobic dancing became a national phenomenon in the 1980s, attracting hordes of participants, especially women. It's still one of the most popular sports around the world.

Think aerobic dancing and you immediately envision quick side-to-side moves, dancing on the balls of the feet, skips, and jumps. This "punishment" requires fit feet in top-notch shape.

Because impact forces from aerobics can reach up to six times the force of gravity transmitted to each of the 26 bones in the foot, shoes with great cushioning, shock absorption, and medial-lateral stability are essential. Feet with excessive pronation or supination may require orthotics.

To accommodate the demands of aerobic dancing, shoes need a good arch design, a thick upper-leather or strap support for forefoot stability and slippage prevention, and a high toe box to

**SMART SOURCES**

*For products helpful in treating sports injuries, visit:*

www.fitnesszone.com/ commercial/

*Fitness Mart online catalog and links:*

http://fitnessmart.com/ priorfit/index.html

*For products to help injured ankles and knees visit:*

Wobbleboard www.kinetichealth.com/ edull.htm.

Active Ankle Trainer www.activeankle.com

prevent nail problems. Double-tie shoes snugly in the toe box to allow toes to spread; tie them tighter around the arch.

## Plantar Fasciitis (Arch Pain)

Arch pain is often caused by frequent stress on the plantar aspect (bottom of the foot) in an aerobics routine. When the plantar fascia—a supportive, fibrous band of tissue running from the heel to the ball of the foot—becomes inflamed, the bottom of the foot hurts. Shoes with proper support in the arch often prevent plantar fasciitis; if not, try a custom orthotic or buy another shoe.

## Heel Spurs

Heel spur syndrome, related to plantar fasciitis, occurs after calcium deposits build up on the underside of the heel bone. Heel spurs form gradually over many months. Both plantar fasciitis and heel spurs can be avoided by a proper warm-up that includes stretching the band of tissue on the bottom of the foot.

## Sesamoiditis

Sometimes referred to as the "ball bearings of the foot," the sesamoids are a set of accessory bones beneath the large first metatarsal bone. Incredible forces are exerted on the sesamoid bones during aerobics, resulting in inflammation and fractures. Proper shoe selection and custom orthotics can help avoid sesamoiditis.

## Shinsplints

Aside from ankle sprains, shinsplints are perhaps the most common injury to the lower body, as the muscles attached to the shinbone bring the foot up and down. The pain is usually an inflammation of the shin muscle and tendon due to stress fractors. Treat shin pain with cold compresses immediately after the workout to reduce inflammation. Proper stretching beforehand and strengthening of muscles will help prevent shinsplints.

## Achilles Tendon and Calf Pain

The frequent rising on the toes during an aerobics routine often creates pain and tightness in the large muscles in the back of the legs, which can create pain and tightness in the calf and inflammation of the Achilles tendon. Again, stretching the calf muscles gently before and after the workout will help alleviate the pain and stiffness.

## Stress Fractures

Probably the most common injuries to aerobics exercisers, stress fractures are caused by poor shoe selection, hard surfaces, and overuse. Women are more likely to develop stress fractures than men, and these injuries usually happen in the lesser metatarsal bones. When swelling and pain surface, see a podiatrist. X-ray evaluation and early treatment can prevent a disabling injury.

## Low Back Pain

Twisting and jumping can cause low back pain, especially if you haven't warmed up sufficiently or have poor abdominal strength. As a precaution, warm up and stretch slowly, cool down properly, and make abdominal exercises an integral part of your training program.

**F.Y.I.**

• Start by exercising twice a week for several weeks, then gradually increase to a maximum of five times a week.

• Do not attempt to exercise through pain, or you may aggravate an acute injury into a chronic or permanent one.

## Preventing Aerobic Dancing Injuries

Most injuries are preventable, especially those resulting from improper shoes, surfaces, or routines, and overuse of muscles through too vigorous a regimen. Here are some tips to keep you dancing:

• Use common sense in selecting an aerobics class. A multi-impact class that allows you to start at a low-impact level and work your way up as your conditioning improves is a wise choice.

• Make sure the teacher—even of an exercise video—is certified. Also be sure the level of the class isn't too advanced.

• Choose floors that are aerobic-dance-friendly, such as hardwood floors with padded mats. Don't do high-impact routines on carpet.

• Avoid ballistic stretching.

# Cycling

## Common Injuries

• Hamstring muscle pulls

• Falls with injuries to head, shoulder, arms, hands, hips, ankles, feet

• Ankle sprains

- Testicular damage

- Pressure injury to the perineum (the area between the vagina and anus)

- Runner's knee

The bicycle was first invented in Europe in the late 1700s. Today, more than 100 million Americans still ride for pleasure on occasion. In New York City alone, 100,000 people use a cycle as a means of transportation to work. Injuries, to say the least, are rather common.

Every day, cyclists sustain overuse injuries from pushing themselves beyond their limitations. As with all athletic injuries, pain that is persistent indicates a need to seek treatment from a sports medicine specialist familiar with cycling injuries.

## Knee Pain

Some intrinsic knee problems like swelling, clicking, or popping should be immediately evaluated by a sports medicine specialist. Cartilage irritation or deterioration, usually under the kneecap, can be caused by a biomechanical imbalance, improper saddle height, or faulty foot positioning on the pedals. Riding in too high a gear, too far uphill, or standing on the pedals may aggravate the problem. Cleated shoes or touring shoes with ribbed soles that limit side-to-side motion can cause knee pain if the knees, feet, and pedals are misaligned.

## Shinsplints

Pain to either side of the leg bone may be caused by muscle or tendon inflammation related to an imbalance between opposing muscle groups in the leg or excessive foot pronation. Proper stretching and corrective orthoses for pronation can help prevent shinsplints.

## Achilles Tendinitis

Irritation and inflammation of the tendon that attaches to the back of the heel bone can be caused by improper pedaling, seat height, lack of a proper warm up, or overtraining. This condition is usually seen in more experienced riders and can be treated with RICE. Chronic pain or swelling should be professionally evaluated.

## Sesamoiditis

Sometimes known as the "ball bearings of the foot," the sesamoids are two small bones found beneath the first metatarsal bones. The sesamoids can inflame or rupture under the stress of cycling. Sesamoiditis can be relieved with proper shoe selection and orthoses.

## Numbness

Impingement of small nerve branches between the second and third or third and fourth toes can cause swelling that results in numbness, tingling, burning, or sharp, shooting pains into the toes. Wider shoes or loosening toe straps or laces can alleviate the problem. If it persists, try a clipless system.

Numbness or tingling with leg pain may represent acute compartment syndrome, a serious problem that requires immediate medical attention.

## Low Back and Knee Pain

These may well be a function of a poor fit, especially in long-distance biking. Have a bike shop check if your bicycle's frame selection, seat height, crank-arm length, and other specifications are right for your size and shape.

## Overuse Injuries

These generally affect the neck, back, and knee and also can be traced to the bike's design, especially seat and handlebars.

# Preventing Cycling Injuries

• Wear protective gear—helmets, eye goggles, padded shorts or pants—and appropriate shoes.

• Stretch the major muscle groups used in cycling—the gluteals, the quadriceps, calves, and hamstrings—before and after getting on the bike.

• Be sure the seat is at the proper height when you're on the bike: knees should be slightly flexed and hips over the knees.

• Start riding slowly and work up to normal rate of pedaling.

• For efficient training, your pulse should be 60 to 70 percent of the maximum.

• Reduce the risk for overuse injuries by frequently varying hand and neck positions.

**SMART MOVE**

You may not think that flexibility is important in injury-free cycling, but it is. "Excessive tightness of the hamstrings or hip flexor muscles affects pelvic positioning on the bike seat, which may contribute to low back pain," says Janeen Hellenbrand, P.T. "Inflexibility of the quadriceps muscle may result in knee irritation."

• Altering positions alleviates neck stress and nerve compression leading to hand weakness.

• Strong abdominal muscles help prevent back pain.

• Drink plenty of water to avoid dehydration.

• Stretching out tight muscles while riding can eliminate stiffness.

• Include a proper warm-up and cooldown in every ride.

# Cycling Shoes

Cycling shoes must have a stable shank to efficiently transfer power from your feet to the pedals. The lack of shank support in sneakers allows the foot to collapse through the arch while pedaling, which may cause arch pain, tendon problems, or burning under the bottom of the foot. A rigid shank can protect your feet from the stress of pedaling.

Investing in a cycling-specific shoe is a good idea if you have had preexisting problems with your feet or wear orthotics. Riders with mild bunions or hammertoes should select a wider, deeper shoe that will accommodate the deformity.

Select a shoe designed for racing and mountain biking. For the casual rider without known foot problems, cross-training shoes provide the necessary support across the arch and instep. They also provide the heel lift that cycling shoes give. Combination cycling-hiking shoes meet the needs of the casual rider well.

## Toe Clips

The use of toe clips and their degree of sophistication separates the casual rider from the devotee. Toe clips range from traditional clips to newer shoe-cleat ensembles—"clipless systems"—resembling ski bindings. Many companies model their units on the French manufacturer Look. A Look-compatible unit will offer the most diverse combinations of shoes and clips from which to choose.

## Biomechanics and Cycling

Biomechanics plays a crucial role in efficient, satisfying cycling. For example, when seated on a bike with hands on the handlebars, the hands, shoulders, and front axle should all be in line.

If, for example, an experienced cyclist's knees hurt after a 30-mile ride, the problem may be a biomechanical imbalance correctable with a prescription orthotic.

# Tennis and Racquet Sports

## Common Injuries

- Ankle sprains

- Plantar fasciitis

- Tennis toe

**SMART DEFINITION**

**Biomechanics**

Biomechanics is the study of external forces on the living body.

- Stress fracture

- Shin splints

- Corns

- Calluses

- Blisters

- Tennis elbow

- Back pain

It doesn't take a superior athlete to play tennis, but care must always be taken to avoid injuries to muscles not vigorously exercised off the court. This is especially true of the foot and ankle, which are put under considerable stress by the continuous side-to-side motion and the quick stopping and starting the sport requires. Different court surfaces also stress the foot and ankle in different ways.

Similar racquet sports, such as racquetball, squash, badminton, and paddle tennis, also leave the foot and ankle susceptible to injury. Injuries common to tennis and other racquet sports include ankle sprains, stress fractures, plantar fasciitis, and tennis toe, among others. If they're minor, some of these injuries are self-treatable; others require the care of a physician to get you back on the court.

## Ankle Sprains

The most common of all tennis injuries, ankle sprains usually occur when the foot turns inward,

# New Hope for Ankle Problems

Athletes need no longer fear the prolonged suffering and debilitating effects of severe ankle sprains.

"Orthopedic surgeons now treat ankle sprains with specialized braces, new reconstruction methods, and arthroscopy techniques, which allow a return to full activity quickly," says Pierce Scranton, M.D., team physician for the Seattle Seahawks professional football team.

Five years ago athletes with severe ankle sprains might be in a cast for six weeks. New braces and ankle wraps combined with aggressive rehabilitation eliminate stiffness and soreness, allowing athletes to return to full activity in about one week. More serious ankle injuries that once required surgery now can be treated with arthroscopy to find bone chips, spurs, and pieces of torn ligament without opening the ankle.

According to Dr. Scranton, ankle arthroscopy has proven particularly useful for athletes with impingement syndrome—painful bone spurs that once required hospitalization, open surgery, and 8 to 10 weeks' rehabilitation.

"With ankle arthroscopy, athletes can be treated as outpatients and return to full activity within two to three weeks."

causing swelling and pain on the outside of the ankle. To self-treat a mild ankle sprain, apply RICE.

## Plantar Fasciitis

Stress on the bottom of the foot sometimes causes arch pain. The plantar fascia, a supportive, fibrous band of tissue running the length of the foot, becomes inflamed and painful. If arch pain persists, consider investing in better shoes, an over-the-counter support or a custom orthotic.

**F.Y.I.**

• In 1996, the number of tennis players increased 3 percent over the previous year.

• Even so, tennis playing was down 9 percent from 1987 to 1996.

• The Tennis Industry Association's "Initiative to Grow the Game" promises to interest more young people in the sport.

## Tennis Toe

A subungal hematoma, or tennis toe, occurs when blood accumulates under the nail. Tennis toe can usually be traced to improper shoes, and should be drained by a podiatrist for quicker recovery. For slight buildup, cool compresses and ice will provide relief.

## Stress Fractures and Shinsplints

Sometimes the long metatarsal bones behind the toes fracture and swell under the stress, causing severe pain when walking. Shinsplints, which are microtears of the anterior calf muscles, and Achilles tendon pulls of the posterior calf muscles are treatable with RICE. These injuries tend to occur on harder court surfaces, and should be fully healed before you resume play. Persistent pain should signal a visit to the doctor.

## Corns, Calluses, and Blisters

Such friction injuries are readily self-treatable, yet care should be taken to ensure that self-treatment does not aggravate the problem. To treat corns and calluses, buff problem areas with a pumice stone after bathing. For blisters, pierce the side with a sterilized needle and drain, then apply an antibiotic cream. Do not remove the roof of the blister. Application of a frictionless pad provides relief from blisters.

## Tennis Elbow

Caused by overuse, tennis elbow or tedinitis is actually an inflammation of the tendon fibers attaching the forearm muscles to the elbow. Certain repetitive motions involved in serving and hitting overhead or backhand shots can provoke the problem. To prevent tendinitis, players must improve their skill so that less stress is put on the wrist and foream. A tennis pro or sports medicine specialist can offer advice.

To relieve pain, give the arm a rest from playing and treat it with RICE. After three days, a series of strengthening exercises should begin.

## Low Back Pain

The sudden twists and turns inherent in racquet sports can really strain your lower back, especially if it's already weak because of prior injury or poor abdominal strength. Here again, strengthening exercises for the back and abs are prescribed, as well as a quick check of posture because many people slouch after playing. This puts the spine in an extreme position, triggering soreness. Stretching can also prevent and alleviate low back pain.

# Choosing a Foot-Friendly Tennis Court

Some courts found these days are harder and more durable. Clay courts, and new crushed stone "fast dry" courts, which duplicate the softness of clay but require less upkeep, are becoming more popular because players can slide on the soft surface. Clay and fast-dry courts are undoubtedly safest to the foot and ankle.

Outdoor courts are often surfaced with asphalt or concrete, and indoor courts with carpet, none of which allow for sliding. It's becoming more popular to coat the harder outdoor courts with a cushioning surface containing rubber granules. While this coating softens the court and slows down the game, it's no more forgiving to the feet than the concrete or asphalt beneath it.

# Buying Tennis Shoes

Regardless of court surface, proper shoes are crucial to injury prevention. Shoes should be specifically designed for tennis. Unlike running shoes, proper tennis shoes "give" enough to allow for side-to-side sliding. Running shoes have too much traction and may cause injury to the foot and ankle. In addition, running shoes don't have padded toe boxes, leading to toe injuries.

Heels should be snug fitting to prevent slipping from side to side, and both heel and toe areas adequately cushioned. The arch should provide soft support, and the toe box needs to have adequate depth to prevent toenail injuries.

# Easing In

All racquet sports require quick acceleration, twisting, and pivoting, putting the whole body under stress. Even if you consider yourself generally healthy, ease into a regular schedule of playing time. Whenever you use a different court, get a "feel" for the new surface before playing a match. Even professional tennis players arrive at tournaments up to a week early to acclimate themselves.

Remember that persistent minor aches and pains are not normal, and will become aggravated if ignored or neglected.

# Golf

## Common Injuries

- Neck or back pain

- Golfer's elbow

- Shinsplints

- Feet pain, blisters

- Muscle pulls and leg strains

Close to 45 million Americans enjoy golf on an amateur level. Above and beyond the satisfaction of competition and enjoying the outdoors, a hilly round of golf affords the opportunity for a four- to five-mile workout that can reduce stress and improve cardiovascular health. However, injuries are common among amateur golfers, with about 65 percent incurring at least one injury.

According to Sarah Weitz, former physical therapist at Meriter Sports Medicine, in Madison, Wisconsin, biomechanical problems in your golf game can result in a wide variety of injuries, which might be avoided by some initial coaching from a pro.

When injured, participation is no substitute for rehabilitation. Injured body parts must be thoroughly treated to meet the hill demands of golf. If you are injured, your return should be gradual. As much as you may want to get back to your game, take it slow. A healthy body makes for a more enjoyable game, and possibly a better scorecard at the end of the day.

**SMART MOVE**

"Good foot action is the mark of an accomplished golfer," points out golf legend Jack Nicklaus. "All timing, distance, and direction comes out of the lower body with the feet leading the way," he says.

First, your weight is placed lightly on the balls of your feet, balanced between your front and rear foot. Then there is a slight shift to the back foot, then another shift back to the front. Sound like dance steps? These intricate movements actually describe what goes on below the knees during an ordinary golf swing.

Nicklaus or any professional will tell you that problems with the feet, even a painful corn or callus, can impede timing and balance to the point that it's reflected on the scorecard at the end of the day.

## Golfer's Elbow, Hand and Wrist Pain

As a result of the pulling action of the left arm as it strikes the ground with force, golfer's elbow manifests itself in tenderness usually experienced in the left inner elbow radiating down the outside of the forearm toward the small pinkie finger. (The fact that most golfers experience pain in the left elbow is related to the large preponderance of right-handed golfers.) The cause is poor swing mechanics and conditioning.

The repetitive stress placed on the left wrist during the swing provokes a chain of inflammation from the wrist tendon where it attaches to the elbow, resulting in tendinitis. The only real way the injury will disappear is to take a break from golf for a bit, treat the elbow with RICE, and begin strengthening exercises for the wrist and elbow.

Wrist pain may also occur in the nondominant hand and can be relieved with rest and strengthening exercises.

## Muscle Pulls and Leg Strains

Failure to warm-up and stretch adequately before playing golf can cause muscle pulls and strains in the lower back, trunk, and calves. The torque of a golf swing itself and the hilly terrain increases the stress, predisposing the golfer to injury.

## Injuries to Feet and Toes

Foot problems affecting golfers—blisters, neuromas (inflamed nerve endings), and other foot pains—are usually brought on by wearing improper shoes.

## Low Back/Neck Pain

"Low back pain is one of the most frequent and occasionally disabling problems in amateur and professional golfers," says Scott A. Banks, Ph.D., Or-

## Good Form! The Swing

Biomechanics play a crucial part in developing the ideal golf swing. The
lateral motion and the pivoting intrinsic to the golf swing can be function-
ally impeded by certain biomechanical conditions. Faulty biomechanics can
inhibit proper foot function, and your game will suffer.

The anatomy of a biomechanically sound swing goes like this: During set-
up, your weight should be evenly distributed on both feet with slightly more
weight on the forefoot as you lean over, and slightly more weight on the insides of both feet.

Maintenance of proper foot alignment on the backswing is critical for
control of the downswing and contact position. During the backswing, weight
should be shifted to the back foot. It should be evenly distributed on the back
foot or maintained slightly on the inside. Shifting weight to the outside leaves
you susceptible to the dreaded "sway," a common error in swing. Without an
exact reversal of the sway in the downswing, swaying will result in improper
contact with the ball.

As the back foot remains in a solid position on the back swing without any
rolling to the outside, the front foot is in turn rolling to the inside. The front
heel occasionally comes off the ground to promote a hill shoulder turn. Com-
pletion of the backswing places the weight on the back foot evenly distributed
between forefoot and rearfoot, with the weight left on the front foot rolling to
the inside.

The downswing involves a rapid shift of weight from back to front foot;
momentum brings the heel of the front foot down, and follow-through naturally causes a rolling of the back foot to the inside and the front foot to the
outside. Golf should always be played from the insides of the feet.

Like the great Nicklaus said, "lively feet" are critical to a successful golf
game. Having healthy, biomechanically stable feet is the first prerequisite for
achieving that goal.

thopedic Research Laboratory, Good Samaritan Medical Center in West Palm Beach, Florida. "Poor swing mechanics, excessive practice, and poor physical conditioning can cause low back pain in recreational golfers. Golfers with right-side, low back pain experience aggravation of their symptoms during the impact of the golf ball through the follow-through phase of their swings. We hypothesize that a golfer's sideways bending combined with an increase in twisting speed contribute to degeneration and injury."

# Preventing Golf Injuries

In golf, it's hard to tell where prevention ends and treatment begins. Certainly many of problems involving the feet and toes can be prevented by buying shoes designed specifically for golf that fit well, along with socks made of synthetic fibers, like acrylic, which maintain their shape without stretching and keep the feet cool, preventing blisters.

• An appropriate, thorough warm-up and a sports-specific stretching program will go a long way toward heading off muscle strains in the legs, trunk, and back. Include hamstring stretches, rotational twists, and lying on the ground with knees to chest as a part of your regimen.

• Strengthening exercises for the wrist and arm will keep golfer's elbow at bay.

• Before teeing off, practice the swing with your short club several times without hitting any balls.

• Then practice hit a couple of dozen balls at about 80 percent of your normal speed.

• Using orthoses will equalize the weight load on the lower extremities and rest overused muscles.

# Basketball

## Common Injuries

• Finger dislocations and fractures

• Stress fractures

• Plantar fasciitis

• Shinsplints

• Achilles tendinitis

• Jumper's knee

• Shoulder dislocations

### Finger Dislocations and Fractures

It doesn't take much to fracture or dislocate a finger playing basketball. Receiving a pass in such a way that it hits the tip of a finger will typically do the job. Ice will get swelling under control. But if the ball also pushes your finger sideways, you may actually dislocate the joint. If your finger looks disfigured, try pulling on it to reset it. Either scenario may result in a broken finger, so it's essential to consult a doctor for a X-ray if pain persists.

**F.Y.I.**

According to the 1998 State of the Industry Report by the Sporting Goods Manufacturers Association (SGMA):

• Basketball is one of the fastest growing sports in America.

• From 1987 to 1994, basketball participation increased 32 percent.

• The number of men aged 35 to 54 playing basketball more than doubled since 1987.

• Female participation increased 23 percent between 1987 and 1994.

## Stress Fractures, Shinsplints

Midair collisions, erratic lunges for a rebound, or scrambles after a loose ball put the entire body under stress, guaranteed to cause injuries. Especially rough on the calf, foot, and ankle, basketball can do significant damage because of the tremendous pressure exerted in jumping and cutting. That's why the right shoes and sport-specific conditioning are so essential. Two distinct types of injury to the lower extremities can occur in basketball: acute injury from a sudden and forceful blow, or chronic injury, which develops slowly and becomes aggravated over an extended period of time.

In basketball, jumping is the operative word. Whether it's leaping up to receive, intercept, or throw, the stress of the movement can strain the calf muscle. To rehabilitate the injury, stop playing for a couple of days, apply ice, and start a program of slow, careful stretches for the calf.

## Jumper's Knee

Basketball players are prone to inflammation of the tendons that attach to the top and bottom of the kneecap. Responsible for helping the leg to straighten, the quadriceps and patellar tendons are apt to become inflamed with repetitive upright jumping. Jumper's knee can be slow to heal because of limited blood supply to the tendons. But if the condition is mild with pain present only during or after play, it might be treated successfully with RICE followed by moist heat 72 hours later.

The biggest challenge to the athlete with jumper's knee is to develop patience. If you return to play too soon, the whole cycle will start again and may lead eventually to surgery.

## Ankle Sprains, Foot Injuries

There's not much you can do to prevent spraining your ankle and other injuries resulting from a jump or a twist while falling. These accidents are likely to result in ankle sprains, torn ligaments, and tendon ruptures. Ankle sprains that don't respond quickly to RICE should be X-rayed to preclude the possibility of a break.

As with other sports, chronic or overuse injuries can be directly traced to improper preparation and poor footwear, worn-out shoes or a biomechanical fault stressing the foot and ankle.

A lot will depend on the surface on which you play. As in aerobic dancing, the safest floor is made of wood because it absorbs shock. Outdoor asphalt courts and those made of concrete pose the greatest possibility of injury to the lower extremities.

## Plantar Fasciitis

The constant pounding that the feet take running across the court can cause heel pain at the attachment of the plantar fascia (the strong tissue that stretches from the heel to the ball of the foot). The problem usually responds to anti-inflammatory medications, RICE, a stretching program, and/or arch supports (often worn for several months).

Other treatments include ice, ultrasound, or occasionally corticosteroid injections. Heel pain often takes months to go away, but rarely requires surgery.

## Achilles Tendinitis

Persistent jumping can cause an inflammation of the Achilles tendon connecting calf muscles to the heel. Pain and swelling are easily treated with anti-

**SMART SOURCES**

American Orthopedic Foot and Ankle Society (AOFAS)
1216 Pine Street
Suite 201
Seattle, WA 98101
(206) 223-1120
www.aofas.org
This website offers invaluable information on preventing ankle and foot injuries.

The American Podiatric Medical Association
www.apma.org
The website contains a variety of quizzes to help you determine your foot health, foot facts and informative articles on foot care and accident prevention.

800-FOOTCARE (800 366-8227) will provide consumers with free literature on a variety of foot-health topics.

inflammatory medications, icing, and stretches such as the runner's stretch to increase tendon flexibility.

## Shoulder Dislocation

You may not think of basketball as a contact sport but it certainly can be. When a player jumps for a shot and is intercepted by an opponent who hits her throwing arm backward, she could wind up with a dislocated shoulder. Such an injury requires manipulation by a physician followed by exercises to strengthen the rotator cuff muscles.

# Preventing Basketball Injuries

• Chronic injuries can be averted with proper conditioning, including weight training, the proper shoes, and good sense on the court.

• Wear high-topped shoes with ankle support and shock absorption. Replace the shoes before the soles become smooth, or before the uppers begin to tear or come apart. Protect feet from blisters by wearing acrylic socks.

• Chronic pain can often be traced to a biomechanical abnormality that is placing undue stress on a particular part of the foot or ankle. Prescription orthotic devices can correct biomechanical imbalances.

• Selective stretching and strengthening programs, shoe modifications, or strapping of the foot and ankle can also correct biomechanical problems. Lower extremity structural problems that often lead to injury include high arches, flat feet, bowlegs, and tight calf muscles.

## Treating Basketball Injuries

• Don't wait until the game is officially over to deal with an injury. Apply RICE immediately.

• With a chronic injury, the key is to reduce activity level in accordance with the severity of the pain, apply RICE, and use anti-inflammatory medications.

• If you still hurt three to five days after an injury, see a doctor.

• When injury to the foot or ankle occurs, the injured part must recover from the acute inflammatory phase of healing. Then, adequate support with shoes or splints and/or tape may be necessary.

• Strengthen the injured part back to its preinjury condition. If not, it will continue to remain weak and predispose the athlete to reinjury.

# Swimming

## Common Injuries

• Rotator cuff tendinitis

• Swimmer's ear

**F.Y.I.**

• Jet ski injuries are most likely to affect the spine.

• "Jumping" waves (maneuvering right into a wave) is highly dangerous

• Injuries to the shoulder and ankle are also likely.

## Rotator Cuff Tendinitis

Those rotator cuff muscles in your shoulders really take a beating when you hit the swimming pool.

The supraspinatus muscle in the rotator cuff group is the one that's injured the most in swimming. Keep it strong with shoulder exercises recommended by a coach or a physical trainer.

## Swimmer's Ear

Long swims can leave behind water trapped in the ear canal, a perfect breeding ground for bacteria swept into the ear from the swimming pool. After a while, sounds become fuzzy and the ear may begin to itch. Swelling, pain, discharge, and tenderness may follow, signaling trouble. If over-the-counter antibiotic drops don't relieve symptoms and discomfort persists for two or three days, see a physician.

Even if you don't swim, you can get swimmer's ear if you perspire a lot or engage in other activities that predispose your ear to accumulating excess water.

The most sensible precaution is to keep the ear as dry as possible by using earplugs, drying the ears thoroughly after bathing, and shaking out any water that's accumulated once you're out of the pool. Pay attention to water quality before going swimming; if the water doesn't look clean, make other plans. Don't go overboard on cleaning your ears; remember that wax in the ear canal is nature's way of protecting the inner sanctum. Used after swimming, over-the-counter eardrops can also help prevent swimmer's ear, but make sure you allow it to drain out of your ear. What you don't want to do is trap the fluid inside the canal so that the precaution becomes an opportunity for infection.

# Preventing Swimming Injuries

• Include shoulder-strengthening exercises in your conditioning program.

• In rehabilitation, concentrate on number of repetitions, rather than weights.

• Don't stint on getting good advice. Poor technique can precipitate injury. So can trying to go too fast.

• If you experience pain, switch to strokes that don't make you feel uncomfortable.

• Fins can be a sore shoulder's best friend, especially when you're going for distance and endurance.

• Skip hand paddles and kickboards because they put increased stress on the shoulders; so does diving.

# Volleyball

## Common Injuries

• Sand toe

• Turf toe

Players of football, soccer, and basketball have helped make "turf toe" a household term since it

**STREET SMARTS**

"The first time I was injured swimming, there was noticeable pain, but I kept going anyway," says Robert Oster, 38, a computer programmer. "After about a month of this, my shoulder just froze up. It was unbearably painful to lift my arm or move my shoulder at all. After seeing a chiropractor and an acupuncturist, six weeks later I started using my arms swimming again. I gradually worked my way up to full use. Two years later, I decided to see a physical therapist after experiencing pain during two practices in a row. She said I had some very tight back muscles that prohibited the shoulder from moving freely through its entire range. Now I do a series of stretches and back-muscle strengthening exercises. I learned that swimming through the pain only makes it worse and recovery time greater."

was first coined in 1976. With the growing popularity of beach volleyball—which made its debut as an Olympic sport at Atlanta in 1996—can "sand toe" be far behind?

A common injury among beach volleyball players, sand toe is similar to turf toe in that it involves a sprain of the first metatarsophalangeal joint, which connects the big toe to the forefoot. But while a turf-toe injury is usually the result of what orthopedists call hyperdorsiflexion (forward bending of the foot), with the forefoot fixed on the ground and the heel raised, sand toe is caused by an impact that causes hyperplantarflexion, or knuckling over of the toe.

The most common scenario for injury, according to AOFAS spokeswoman Carol Frey, M.D., an orthopedic consultant to the American Volleyball Professionals, involves a running approach from a jump serve or a spike. The injury can also occur when the athlete strikes a firm, nongiving divot in the playing surface, with the weight of the body driving the foot into the sand.

Frey, who conducted a recent retrospective study of 12 cases of sand-toe injuries sustained by professional beach volleyball players, noted that the injury can result in significant functional disability, with push-off, forward drive, running, and jumping all compromised.

Surgery is rarely indicated for sprains of the toe joints, Frey says. Athletes suffering a sand-toe injury should be treated conservatively with taping (to protect the toe from excessive motion), non-steroidal anti-inflammatory medications, shoe wear modification, ice, and rest. After the inflammatory period has passed, toe exercises are recommended to strengthen the intrinsic muscles and promote toe power.

The average player in the study took six months to fully recover. The most effective treatment was taping the involved toe.

Frey noted that beach volleyball players generally do not wear shoes, which would most likely prevent the vast majority of sand-toe injuries.

Court volleyball palyers are likely to suffer the same injuries as basketball players, because both sports require more quickstep reactions from a stationary position. If you play court volley ball, buy a shoe specific to the sport. You'll find they're similar to basketball shoes except that they're lighter, have less midsole support, and a "tighter" sole more responsive to quick starts and stops.

# Winter Sports: Skiing and Ice Skating

## Common Winter Sports Injuries

- Frostbite

- Ankle sprains

- Achilles tendinitis

- Plantar fasciitis

- Blisters

- Neuromas

## WHAT MATTERS, WHAT DOESN'T

*Frostbite*

### What Matters

• People with a history of frostbite often have it recur in the same place.

• In frostbite, skin color changes from blue to whitish.

• A feeling of burning or numbness can indicate frostbite.

• The warming qualities of battery-powered heated ski boots and new exothermic packs help prevent frostbite.

### What Doesn't

• Not seeing the frostbite; other symptoms will indicate its presence.

• Massaging frostbiten body parts. Rubbing may cause additional skin damage.

• Subungal hematoma

Winter athletics bring thrills and challenges unique to ice, snow, high altitude, and cold. The high speeds attained on skis and skates make for exhilarating sports, but they also expose the body to injuries.

Healthy feet and ankles, which act together as accelerators, steering, brakes, and shock absorbers in winter sports, are not only crucial to success in competition, but also help keep the body upright and out of the emergency room. Any problems with the foot or ankle could have serious repercussions for winter-sports participants.

In skiing, particularly at an intermediate or advanced level, the high speeds place tremendous levels of impact trauma on the lower extremities, especially on steep and bumpy runs.

Skating also puts tremendous stress on the ankle. Even casual figure skating requires quick turns and stops negotiated by the lower extremities.

If any preexisting foot conditions, such as corns, calluses, bunions, plantars warts, or hammertoes are present, see a physician for evaluation before buckling or lacing up. A medical examination is also important if you have any preexisting circulatory problems, such as Raynaud's disease or diabetes.

## Blisters

Friction in winter-sports footwear often causes blisters. Do not pop a small blister, but if it breaks on its own, apply an antiseptic and cover with a sterile bandage.

# Ski Boots and Skates

According to the APMA, ski boots and ice skates are the single most important factor in safe and successful skiing and skating. The right fit—snug but not too tight—can prevent injury due to pressure exerted by the constant forward motion and lateral movement of skiing and the quick turns of skating.

Ski boots are available in a forward-entry variety, a rear-entry style for easier entry and more comfort, or "hybrids," which incorporate both designs. Modern systems of cables and buckles make it possible to alter the boots to a near-perfect fit.

Ice skates do not come in as many shapes and sizes. Common side-to-side wobbling in the heel area can be remedied with "shims," or pads, in the heel. Shims can also be added to the counter area, or middle of the skate, for a more snug fit.

Cross-country ski shoes look more like a bicycle shoe than a downhill ski boot. Bound to the ski only at the ball of the foot, cross-country boots should not irritate the balls of the feet.

If you use custom orthoses, insert them into skis and skates. Skiers with minor biomechanical imbalances may encounter a frustrating phenomenon known as "edging."

Ski boots and skates can be "canted" internally to adjust the relationship between the boot and leg. For cases of rolling-in of the foot, or rolling-out caused by flat feet or high arches, cants may be applied directly to the skis or within the boot. This improves edging and enhances performance and control, making the sport safer and more enjoyable.

## Neuromas

Enlarged benign growths of nerves between the toes, neuromas are caused by friction in tight footwear and can result in pain, burning, tingling, or numbness. Neuromas require professional treatment, including an evaluation of skates and boots.

**SMART DEFINITION**

**Edging**

In skiing, edging occurs when the ski rolls to the inside or outside edge, inhibiting the skier's control.

## Sprains and Strains

The stresses of skiing and skating can result in sprains and strains of the foot and ankle. They can be treated with RICE, but medical attention is required for persistent pain.

## Subungal Hematoma

Pressure in the toe box of a ski or skate can cause bleeding under the toenail known as a subungal hematoma. Such a condition should be treated by a physician before the condition worsens to prevent the loss of a toenail.

## Bone Problems

Bunions and tailor's bunions, bony prominences at the joints on the inside or outside of the foot, often become irritated in ski boots or skates. Pain at these joints may indicate a need for a wider or better-fitting boot. Other preexisting conditions, such as hammertoes and plantars warts, and Haglund's deformity (a bump on the back of the heel) can be irritated by an active winter sports regimen. If pain persists, see a doctor. Fractures caused by trauma require immediate medical attention.

# Preventing Winter Sports Injuries

• The right clothing is essential to keep you warm and dry playing winter sports. To protect your skin against moisture, the layer closest to your skin should be made of cotton. The outer layer should be waterproof. If you do get wet and cold, go indoors immediately to change clothing and warm up.

•  For your feet, choose acrylic fiber socks or those made of blends that can handle perspiration effectively. If you get your feet snow-soaked, you could be at risk for frostbite that can actually cost you your toes.

•  Mittens keep hands warmer than gloves because fingers touching each other generate additional heat.

•  To prevent wind on wet skin and clothing, start by playing into the wind and return with the wind at your back.

•  Stretch muscles before taking to the slopes or skating out into the rink. That's the smart way to prevent muscle pulls and tears, and prepare the muscles for the flexing required by the constant "forward lean" stress of skiing and skating.

•  To ski in top form, it's important to keep the ankle perpendicular to the ground and straight up and down while skiing.

•  To prevent injury, always stretch before getting out on your skis; otherwise, the constant up-and-down heel motion of the sport may cause Achilles tendinitis and plantar fasciitis.

# Roller and In-Line Skating

## Common Skating Injuries

- Wrist injuries and fractures

- Cuts, scrapes, and bruises

- Head injuries

- Injuries to the knees and elbows

In-line skating participation has soared, up 859 percent in the last decade, says an American Sports Data study. More than 29 million Americans over age six went in-line skating one or more times in 1997, a 29 percent increase from 1995. And manufacturers' sales of in-line skates and accessories were $520 million in 1997. Whether your skating of choice is roller or in-line, the nature of the activity—with its outdoors arena, fast movement on hard surfaces, and uncontrollable outside factors—makes this one sport with high a risk for participant injury.

## Preventing Skating Injuries

- Wear a helmet and knee and elbow pads to cushion against falls on cement.

- Wear wrist guards as well, although these won't

make skaters invulnerable to fractures. While wrist guards may protect against scrapes and cuts, they are found to be ineffective in preventing many wrist fractures and other serious injuries. Nonetheless, a little protection is far better than none.

• Learn how to fall, so that an outstretched arm and hand don't take the brunt of the tumble.

• Learn how to stop and anticipate obstacles. Be alert to traffic, steep downgrades, and what's around the next bend.

## THE BOTTOM LINE

Mistakes in form add to the probability of being injured. Unless corrected, repeated stress on muscles and joints that aren't sufficiently strong can trigger overuse injuries that will continue to sideline you after symptoms have disappeared. It isn't enough to treat the symptoms: before getting back in the game it's imperative to get advice from a professional on preventing repeat injuries. Embark on a strengthening program and correct faulty technique to prevent further injury.

Playing in cold conditions presents unique challenges and strains due to the need for proper warming up.

Your gear is a major factor in protecting against injury. Wear protective helmets, goggles, and pads; socks made of synthetic fibers; well-fitting athletic shoes; and climate appropriate clothing.

# CHAPTER 7

# Women and Middle-Aged Athletes

## THE KEYS

• Anatomy may be destiny when it comes to the prevalence of certain types of injuries in female athletes.

• This prevalence of injuries is due largely to poorly constructed athletic equipment that have not taken into account women's unique biomechanics.

• Pregnant women can safely participate in sports—even jogging—as long as they observe guidelines issued by the American College of Obstetrics and Gynecology (ACOG).

• To take the guess-work out of selecting a properly fitting sports bra, the American Council on Exercise (ACE) has issued a set of helpful guidelines.

Only a few decades ago, sports were predominately a male pastime with equipment—and particularly athletic shoes—designed exclusively for their anatomy. Because women's unique biomechanics were not considered in the design, they were predisposed to a variety of injuries. Well, all that's changing now with more and more manufacturers offering equipment designed by women for women.

Also on the plus side, more middle-aged and older people are taking up sports or switching sports than ever before. While this is indeed exciting, would-be athletes must be careful not to expect their athletic prowess to return overnight to what it was at their fitness peak. With proper sport-specific conditioning, getting back in the game at any age can be remarkably rewarding and safe.

# Women Athletes

In the 1990s women received more recognition for their tremendous athletic achievements than ever before: In 1995 Nike introduced the first female "signature" basketball shoe (named for Sheryl Swoopes). Since 1996 two new women's professional basketball leagues have been created. And in 1998 Team USA won the first-ever Olympic gold medal awarded for women's hockey.

As deserving as this attention is, it doesn't underscore the one fundamental fact of the sports worlds: women and men are profoundly different.

# Anatomy Is Sports Destiny

• Men have leg lengths that average 56 percent of their total height. Women, on the other hand, have leg lengths that average just 51 percent of their total height.

• Females have wider pelvises, narrower shoulders, and are also more knock-kneed.

• Male athletes have larger lungs and hearts, and higher blood pressure.

• Women athletes have less muscle mass, more body fat, and less ability to mobilize and use oxygen for aerobic metabolism.

• Women have smaller bones and smaller joints.

The accelerated rate of improvement in female athletic records in recent years has prompted predictions that women's performance may someday equal or surpass that of men.

"Unlikely," says Carol Frey, M.D., AOFAS spokeswoman and orthopedic consultant to the Los Angeles Roadrunners and the L.A. Marathon. "Women and men simply aren't on a level playing field because females are, on average, physiologically disadvantaged in comparison with men when it comes to anaerobic and aerobic performance. However, wider pelvises and shorter legs do give females a lower center of gravity, an advantage in sports that require balance, such as gymnastics."

Physiological differences may also explain why women seem more prone to certain types of injuries. A recent University of Washington study of high school athletes, for example, indicated that

**F.Y.I.**

Louisville Slugger offers nine different gloves and mitts "designed by and exclusively for" women playing fast-pitch softball.

girls' cross-country running has the highest rate of injury compared to any other high school sport, including football. Among the female runners studied, one-third had suffered some type of injury, with stress fractures and ankle sprains topping the list. One factor related to this statistic is the shorter female stride, which means more foot strikes per unit of distance than male runners. More impact per mile ultimately leads to more injuries per mile.

# Women and Injuries

But the relationship between anatomical differences and injury vulnerability doesn't stop there. Case in point—tennis elbow, ACL injuries, and kneecap pain are all the result of smaller size and lesser strength, wider hips, narrower bones, hormonal changes, and the way in which one body part aligns with another.

## Tennis Elbow

Women whose tennis racquet is too heavy for their size and strength may be at increased risk of developing tennis elbow. "This can cause them to grip the racquet very tightly, leading to tennis elbow," says Peter Francis, Ph.D., director of the Biomechanics Laboratory at San Diego State University. Women prone to this condition might see if switching to a lighter racquet helps.

## Anterior Cruciate Ligament Injuries

The knee is a woman athlete's Achilles' heel. Female athletes incur two to eight times more anterior cruciate ligament (ACL) injuries than men, particularly female basketball and soccer players.

Just why women are particularly vulnerable to ACL injuries appears to be related to several issues. "The problem is very complicated, and no one factor seems to stand out more than any other," says Bernie Bach, M.D., spokesman for the American Orthopaedic Society for Sports Medicine and director of the Sports Medicine Department at Rush Presbyterian—St. Luke's Medical Center in Chicago.

One possible explanation is the effect of estrogen on the cellular metabolism of the ACL. According to a recent study by Ed Wojtys, M.D., professor of orthopedic surgery at the University of Michigan, women have more ACL injuries during the ovulatory phase of their menstrual cycle. Because the presence of estrogen is greatest during this phase, the researchers think that estrogen fluctuations are a factor in ACL injuries. Finally, a woman's thighbone is narrower than a man's, a factor that somehow increases risk of ACL injury.

"Women athletes beware, " says Laurie Huston, M.S., a research engineer in the Orthopedic Surgery Section. "They are much more likely than male athletes to experience a rupture or tear of their ACL. This is one of the most common knee injuries, but also one of the most devastating."

What clinicians call "rupturing the ACL" is known colloquially as "blowing out" the knee, and involves the tearing of the ligament that runs behind the kneecap, roping the thighbone to the shinbone and stabilizing the kneecap. Once this "rope" is torn, the knee tends to slip and slide.

Huston and Wojtys believe this susceptibility is due to anatomic differences in women such as wider hips, which place greater pressure on the in-

## SMART MOVE

"Ironically, if you study the injury statistics, there really are many more similarities between male and female anatomy than we thought," says Peter Francis, Ph.D., director of the Biomechanics Laboratory at San Diego State University. "Many of the injuries that seem to be more prevalent in women really are nongender specific and can occur with the same frequency in men who have broader hips. What actually may be influencing the injury rate is that women participate in activities like skiing with male partners who are more experienced and skillful. When they try to keep up with them, they naturally become injured."

side of the knee; looser joints, perhaps due to the presence of the hormone relaxin; and less leg strength. But the most serious problem is in the "recruitment order" of knee muscles—who's on top, so to speak, in the rapid-fire progression by which muscles around the knee tighten to stabilize the knee.

In men, the hamstrings (muscles behind the knee) tighten first, followed by the quadriceps (muscles in the front of the thigh). But in women, it's just the other way around and that weakens the knee. This fault may actually be a function of improper training as women work the quadriceps more in weight training than the hamstrings.

# Retraining Is Key

"Women may be predisposed to knee injuries because they're more likely to have a larger Q angle—the alignment of the quadriceps in respect to the kneecap," says Francis. "Broader hips can cause the pull of their quads to be more sideways than it is in men, leading to a condition called chondromalacia patella [wear and tear on the cartilage on the back of the knee]."

To compensate in order to prevent injury, Francis suggests exercises to strengthen the vastus medialis muscle on the inner side of the knee joint. "This muscle creates a tug-of-war situation that could pull the patella back into normal alignment if it's sufficiently strengthened," he explains. To strengthen this muscle, do half squats on one foot. Bend your knees at no more than a 90-degree angle and stand up with your weight on one foot. Alternatively, try sitting on the floor with a towel rolled up behind your kneecaps. Extend your leg so that the heel comes two to three inches off the ground. This will contract the quads and work the muscle. Try performing two sets of 12 reps twice a day.

# Running Risks Caused by Anatomy

The female anatomy is also implicated in triggering knee problems that affect runners. "The wider pelvis and greater angle of the knee make women runners more prone to developing kneecap pain," says AOSSM spokeswoman Etty Griffin, M.D., an orthopedic surgeon and team physician for Agnes Scott College. "As the knee bends and straightens, the knee cap runs up and down in a groove in the femur or thigh bone. Its position in this groove is determined in part by the pull of the quadriceps muscle, which helps straighten out the knee when it contracts."

The way to balance the development of the quadriceps is to strengthen the inner thigh muscles. Recommended exercises are cross-training with cycling and leg lifts. Quadriceps and hamstring stretches to keep the muscles supple are also essential. The AOSSM recommends a hamstring stretch done on the floor sitting with both legs extended out front. Bend one leg so that the heel is flat on the floor, and then grasp the ankle of the straight leg, slowly stretching out the muscles in the back of the leg. To stretch the quads, stand up and bend one leg, leaning backward slightly and grasping the ankle of the bent knee and slowly stretching. This stretch will be felt in the front of the thigh.

## SMART SOURCES

The following sources offer additional information on pregnancy, exercise, and sports:

Fit Maternity & Beyond
P.O. Box 873
Mt. Shasta, CA 96067
(530) 938-4530
www.fitmaternity.com

National Women's
   Health Network
514 10th Street, N.W.
Washington, D.C.
   20004
(202) 628-7814

Motherwell Maternity
   Health and Fitness
1106 Stratford Dr.
Carlisle, PA 17013
(717) 258-4641

Women whose feet roll in while running are at additional risk for kneecap injuries because this pronation causes the kneecap to track to the outside. An easy way to control the pronation and protect injury to the kneecap is to be fitted with arches or supports in your shoes.

# Pregnancy and Sports

One of the best things a woman can do for herself and her baby during pregnancy is to exercise aerobically. According to a study "Exercising Through Your Pregnancy," by James F. Clapp III, M.D., which compared the health of pregnant women who exercised with those who didn't, exercisers had a more upbeat outlook, gained less weight, had fewer complications, and less fetal distress during labor and delivery. They also had shorter labors and deliveries, fewer cesareans, and a faster recovery.

According to the American College of Obstetrics and Gynecology (ACOG), if you're going to exercise stick to it on a regular schedule. Exercising at least three times a week is preferable to intermittent activity.

What you don't want to do is engage in competitive or racquet sports, those that involve ballistic movements (jerky, bouncy motions), or perform deep flexion or extension of joints, says ACOG. Jumping, jarring motions, and rapid changes in direction should be avoided because of joint stability. So should sports that put you at high risk for falling. What types of sports are best for you and baby? Nonweight-bearing sports like swimming, stationary cycling, and walking.

After the baby is born, it isn't smart to try to

rush back into resuming pre-pregnancy levels of exercise. The physiological changes related to pregnancy persist some four to six months post-partum.

Of course, playing sports isn't appropriate for all pregnant women. According to ACOG, sports and exercise should be avoided if any of the following are present:

- Pregnancy-induced high blood pressure

- Preterm rupture of membranes

- Preterm labor during the prior or current pregnancy or both

- Incompetent cervix

- Persistent second or third trimester bleeding

## Running and Pregnancy

The surprising news for pregnant women who are avid runners is that it's okay to continue the sport during pregnancy. According to a 1990 study by the Melpomene Institute, a nonprofit organization that publishes research fitness and health for women, running is safe within certain guidelines. Of the 195 pregnant women in the study, the women were running an average of about 25 miles a week before they got pregnant, and all delivered healthy babies though almost 20 percent had cesarean sections.

Much of the advice is common sense. Because of hormonal changes during pregnancy, particularly of relaxin—which, as its name implies, relaxes

**SMART MOVE**

"Urinary frequency, one of the early signs of pregnancy, is a challenge for expectant runners," says Joan Marie Butler, R.N.C., C.N.M., in her book *Fit & Pregnant: The Pregnant Woman's Guide to Exercise.* "For running, you need to devise some strategic plans. Don't cut back on your fluids . . . you need to stay well hydrated. Plan your runs around a bathroom stop instead."

# Exercise and Pregnancy

Guidelines from the American College of Obstetrics and Gynecology (ACOG) on exercising during pregnancy:

• Pregnant women should avoid exercising in hot, humid weather.

• Expectant mothers should be particularly careful to avoid dehydration, drinking lots of fluid before, during, and after playing. Those who have not been physically active prior to pregnancy should begin with very low intensity levels of exercise, progressing very gradually.

• Pregnancy is not the time to start a weight training program.

• Keep exertion to about 140 beats per minute (70 percent of maximum heart rate).

• After the first trimester, women should avoid exercise positions in which they're lying down, face upward because it will direct cardiac output away from the uterus.

• Prolonged periods of motionless standing should also be avoided.

• Expectant mothers should not exercise to exhaustion and should stop when fatigued.

• Diet during pregnancy should be shored up to include an additional 300 calories daily; active women must consume even more.

• Keep body temperature cool by wearing appropriate clothing, drinking adequate fluids, and exercising in an optimal environment.

ligaments—joints and ligaments are more easily injured. Stretching slowly and thoroughly before and after running will help decrease chances of becoming hurt.

Here are some tips to make running safe for both you and your future athlete:

• Realize that your goals have now changed. Because you're running to remain fit and healthy, take things slowly, don't go for distance, and cut yourself some slack if you just don't feel like running one day.

• If you experience Braxton-Hicks contractions (rhythmic tightening in your lower abdomen), stop and walk until they disappear.

• Buy a good sports bra to keep stress off swollen breasts.

• Pay attention to terrain. The new you is a lot more ungainly, and falling is easier because of changes in gait.

• Modify your workout immediately upon learning you're pregnant. That means no racing or hard, long runs.

• Consult your doctor about how much running is good for you once you hit the second and third trimesters.

• Stop running immediately if you feel persistent contractions, fatigue, faint, leakage, or anything that seems different from normal. See your doctor for an evaluation.

• As you advance in your pregnancy consider exercises like cycling, swimming, walking, cross-country skiing, and low-impact aerobics, which are less weight bearing.

• If you didn't run before you became pregnant, don't start now.

# Women's Sporting-Goods Equipment

Women athletes are finally coming into their own. Not only are more women getting professional recognition and product endorsements, but manufacturers of sporting-goods equipment are also sitting up and finally beginning to take notice. The market for female athletic gear is growing, and consumers want products designed with their specific needs in mind. And they're starting to get it in a big way.

"The industry now recognizes that women need different products from men, but ones that offer the same technical benefits, such as moisture and temperature control," says Ellen Wessel, president of Moving Comfort and chair of SGMA's Sports Apparel Products Council. "Instead of downsizing men's apparel, manufacturers are focusing very specifically on women's needs for comfort, fit, and performance. This means they are producing garments for narrower backs, shorter arms, broader hips, narrower waists, and longer rises from the groin to the waist."

## Buying the Right Sports Bra

A woman's regular everyday bra is no more appropriate for playing sports than a pair of running shoes is for tennis, aerobic dancing, or cycling. Yet knowing which sports bra is best for your figure can be difficult to determine. Here are some recommendations from the American Council on Exercise (ACE) and other experts:

• Compression bras are the best choice for smaller busts because tissue is flattened against the

# Do Sports Bras Really Deliver?

A recent study by the American Council on Exercise (ACE) found that many top-selling sports bras offer little more comfort and support than everyday ones. In order to educate women about the choices available, ACE researchers led by John Porcari, M.D., of the University of Wisconsin, La Crosse, evaluated five of the most popular sports bras designed for large-breasted women (size C-cup or larger). These included Athena's Moving Comfort ($38); Champion's Action Shape Sports Top ($36); Champion's Sports Shape ($25); Danskin's Support Contour ($30), and Hanes Sports' Level 3, Racer Back ($11). Here's what they found:

• The Champion AS, Champion SS, Hanes, and Danskin bras were all significantly more comfortable than the Athena bra.

• The Champion AS, Athena, and Champion SS allowed less vertical movement than the Hanes and Danskin bras.

• The Champion AS, Athena, and Champion SS provided about equal support, which was significantly more than the Hanes and Danskin brands.

• The Hanes and Danskin bras did not provide any greater support than the participants' daily bras.

• The bra rated highest by women in the study for biomechanical construction, comfort, and support was Champion's Action Shape Sports Top.

• The Athena bra was rated lowest in comfort.

chest. Larger breasts get better support in a harness-type construction that encapsulates each breast.

• When trying on a bra, mimic the motions you'd do in a sport in order to see whether it offers sufficient support.

**SMART SOURCES**

Sporting Goods Manu-
facturers Association
200 Castelwood Drive
North Palm Beach, FL
33408-5696
(561) 842-4100
www.sportlink.com/
sport

SGMA conducts annual
surveys on sports
participation, along
with studies on a
variety of subjects
including women and
sports.

• To prevent chaffing due to poor ventilation, look for new fabrics such as CoolMax and Nike's DriFit.

• Choose a bra with nonstretch straps that are wide and don't slip, and check out the possible advantages of a Y-back design.

• Look for wide armholes that won't cut into the underarm, padded seams, a wide back panel to support the back, and covered hooks.

• A back closure will help prevent irritation and be more secure and less likely to open suddenly.

## The Right Shoe and the Right Fit to Avoid Injuries

Women's athletic shoes didn't come into their own until recently. For years, women have had to make do with shoes and other equipment originally designed for men but scaled down to accommodate women's smaller size. That just hasn't worked.

"Although women represent a major portion of the athletic-shoe market, many female runners complain about the difficulty of finding comfortable running shoes," Carol Frey says. "The irony is that most women's running shoes aren't women's shoes, but merely smaller versions of men's shoes. The lasts (shoe forms) are built according to men's feet, and therefore the shoes are actually made for male athletes."

Taking men's shoes and scaling down key internal dimensions is not usually effective because women's feet are shaped differently from men's, especially at the heel. Due to physiological differences, female runners generally complete the heel-toe gait faster and strike the ground more often to cover the same distance, Frey points out. Because women typically pronate more than men, they need shoes that include control features such as increased firmness in the medial heel area, medial internal heel wedge, straighter last, and a strong medial heel counter.

"The majority of female foot problems that physicians encounter result from improper shoewear," says Frey. "The same industry that has provided improperly fitting dress shoes is also responsible for the lag in the production of adequate athletic shoewear for women."

While manufacturers now offer an increasing array of shoes designed for women, just how well they will sell appears to be a question mark. "Women have been buying men's sports equipment for years, so there is still some resistance in the marketplace to women-specific products," says Lisa Kantor, product manager for Fila, in *Gaining Ground,* a 1998 progress report on women and sports by SGMA. "Manufacturers and retailers have to wonder if the product is really necessary from a business perspective. Are we simply cannibalizing men's business? Will women think the product is inferior because it's targeted at women?"

Kantor's concern that women-specific products have a negative connotation is shared by others in manufacturing, and for good reason. "I think for years women's products were inferior to men's," says Sue Levin, women's brand director at Nike. "They carried a lower price point and were color-ups of men's products. But that's ended. We are designing for women with the help and advice of women athletes. It's making a difference. Nike has had annual double-digit sales growth in women's footwear for the last four years."

## Women's Ski Equipment

Similar concerns have been voiced about women's ski equipment. In her book *Women Ski,* Claudia Carbone strongly criticized the manufacturers of ski equipment for putting women at risk of injury because of failure to incorporate their unique physique in design specs. "Ski equipment has always been designed for men," she says. "They are usually taller, stronger, have longer legs, and a higher center of mass. Equipment that is ideal for men may be terrible for women."

What's a skiing woman to do? Some pointers:

• To be sure that skis are the right weight and flexibility, buy those that have an "L" designation.

• To safely control skis, women need boots that are softer and more flexible around the ankles. Raichle and Salomon design liners and shells for women.

• To avoid distorting your boots' fit don't tuck in ski pants or wear heavy socks.

# The Middle-Aged Athlete

Midlifers and seniors are getting into sports in record numbers. A 1996 study examined trends in seven areas—aerobics, bicycling, calisthenics, walking, running, swimming, and exercising with equipment—over a two-year period between 1993 and 1995. Here's what it found:

• More seniors became involved in sports and exercise than any other group with 17 percent of adults over 65 taking up these activities.

• Pre-retirees were next with 15 percent more adults between the ages of 55 to 64 playing.

• Less than 1 percent of those aged 25 to 34 got into sports in the same period.

• Between 1993 and 1995, the number of adults over age 25 who played sports or exercised at least six times a year increased by 6.6 million.

• A third of this group reported engaging in one of the seven activities studied at least twice a week.

• More women (55.4 million) than men (43.4 million) took part in the sports and fitness activities studied.

More Americans than ever before seem to be paying attention to advice from the U.S. Surgeon General regarding the health benefits of sports and exercise.

"This trend is very encouraging," says John Lucas, Ph.D., professor emeritus of kinesiology at Pennsylvania State University, and former long-distance runner in the 1952 Olympics. "But my concern is that middle-aged people taking up sports for the first time have the attitude that 'I'll get to it whenever I have the time.' That simply doesn't work. Not only is it a waste of energy to play on the occasional weekend, but it's almost a guarantee of becoming injured."

Lucas, who at 72 is still an avid runner, says that the correct prescription for midlifers just getting

**F.Y.I.**

Most Popular Sports for Seniors (age 55+)

• Fitness walking
• Treadmill
• Stationary bike
• Golf
• Bowling
• Camping
• Free weights
• Freshwater fishing
• Resistance machine
• Tennis

*Source:* Sporting Good Manufacturers Association

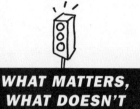

## WHAT MATTERS, WHAT DOESN'T

**For Middle-Aged Athletes:**

## What Matters

• Engaging in strength-building activities to prevent falls that experts say result from fractures.

• Warming up before you stretch in order to avoid tearing muscles and straining ligaments.

• Preparing your body to change sports by engaging in a sport-specific conditioning program.

## What Doesn't

• Cross-training in several activities that work the same muscle groups.

• Trying to improve balance to avoid falling. Balance is inherited and doesn't change after the preteen years.

into sports is to make a commitment to participate 200 times a year. "If you do it less frequently, there will be no appreciable quantitative effects on your body or your skill level," he says. "You just might as well stay at home and watch reruns of *I Love Lucy.*"

Making a transition from a sedentary lifestyle to becoming involved in recreational athletics or changing from one sport to another must be done with extreme slowness and care. "At midlife, the best way to prevent injury is to increase just one variable—endurance, time, or intensity by just 5 percent every other month," Lucas says. "Start off very modestly with about 30 minutes of activity and chronicle what you've done, how long you've done it, and what your pulse rate was in a diary. By the end of a year, you will have accomplished something substantial."

Key to proper training is learning how to take your pulse for an accurate measure of your heart rate. "The best place to measure your pulse is one and one-half inches (about the length of your thumb) below your wrist where you can see your veins," says Lucas. "With four fingers, press lightly on your skin so that you feel both the strong and weak beat. If you've been a nonathlete, you should work at a maximum pulse rate of between 100 and 110 beats per minute. As the weeks go by and your heart gets stronger, gradually work up to 115. Getting into sports and becoming fit must be done scientifically if it's going to be done safely."

# New Skills for Familiar Sports

Picking up that old tennis racquet you used when you were a high school star is exciting. But while it's tempting to think your prowess will return as soon as you step back on the court, lots has changed since the days you lettered. Take the guidelines concerning how to keep your body sufficiently hydrated during sports. At one time, water breaks were tightly scheduled, and water was even somewhat salted. Today, nutritionists and sports medicine physicians have re-evaluated the importance of drinking adequate amounts of liquid during workouts. What, when, and how much you should drink has practically become a science of its own (see chapter 1).

So too has theory changed regarding strategies to prevent injuries. For example, researchers now have better insight as to who should have a pre-sport physical before getting back into the game; the psychological profile of the frequently injured athlete; the domino effect of the second injury syndrome, etc. Coaches, for example, now know that supporting your racquet with two hands playing backhand will minimize risk of hurting your back. Dermatologists now advise golfers to consider wearing two gloves so that the right hand doesn't age prematurely from the otherwise unequal sun exposure. Learning how to fall in order to protect your wrists and fingers from injury in sports like cycling, skiing, and skating decreases your chances of being sidelined. Finally, knowing how to recognize which injuries need simple first-aid care and which require immediate medical attention can make your re-entry into the world of sports a delight rather than a catastrophe.

The bottom line is that it makes smart sport sense to spruce up your skills and knowledge by taking some coaching or enrolling in classes before plunging back into all-out play.

## SMART MOVE

"Be realistic in your goal of getting back to the same level of competency you had when you played high school or college sports," says Peter Francis, Ph.D., director of the biomechanical laboratory at San Diego State University. "A sensible formula to follow is to allow one month of training for every year you've been inactive. If you've been out of the game for ten years, give yourself ten months to get back where you were. That way you'll sidestep overuse and other injuries."

# Changing Sports

Just because your muscles are trained to cut through water smoothly and aggressively doesn't mean your musculoskeletal structure will be equally conditioned for jogging or other sports. "The big mistake athletes make is assuming that fitness is transferable from one sport to another," says Lee Rice. "Because they jog 25 to 50 miles a week, they think they can go out for basketball at a similar intensity, and they wind up pulling a hamstring because they're not in shape for basketball."

Recreational athletes who want to cross-train or switch sports entirely need to observe the law of specificity by training those muscles that are under high demand in a new activity. "The principle is similar to that of transforming yourself from someone who's sedentary to an athlete," says Rice. "Begin training at very low intensity levels, conditioning the muscles that will be used in the new sport. That means reproducing the movements and skills involved in the new activity in your warm-up and conditioning program. You must build up duration, frequency, and intensity slowly and carefully by applying the 10 percent a week rule to each variable until you've attained your performance goals. Using this principle, you should be fully competitive in a new sport within four to six weeks, and you will have minimized chances of hurting yourself!"

The good news is that cross-training actually decreases injury level. In a study that compared injuries among triathletes with marathon runners, researchers discovered that triathletes had fewer injuries because they do more than one activity at a time, varying the biomechanical stress on muscle groups.

# Headaches, Exercise, and Heart Disease

In people whose headaches begin after age 50, as well as in those with risk factors for heart disease, head pain that begins during exercise and disappears with rest could indicate heart disease. "In these types of headaches, the pain occurs in the head instead of in the chest," warns neurologist Richard Lipton, M.D., codirector of the Headache Unit at Montefiore Medical Center in the Bronx, New York.

"Although most headaches associated with exercise are benign, people with 'cardiac headaches' may not experience other signs of heart disease," Lipton says. Though he suspects the condition is rare, he's unsure of how frequently the diagnosis is overlooked. "That's because most physicians and the public are unaware of the possible link between exercise headaches and heart disease," he says.

Because of the potentially serious consequences, athletes who experience headaches triggered by exertion should consult their physician. Such exertional headaches require careful evaluation.

"The reassuring news is that by correctly diagnosing cardiac headaches we have a tremendous opportunity to treat heart disease and prevent heart attacks," says Lipton.

One of the key factors in diagnosing cardiac headaches is the ability to distinguish them from migraine. The danger is that many migraine medications could actually exacerbate the condition of a cardiac headache by constricting the coronary arteries.

**SMART DEFINITION**

**Cardiac headaches**

Head pain that coincides with exercise onset. This could signal silent heart disease, especially if rest appears to resolve the headache.

**THE BOTTOM LINE**

Women's athletics is coming of age: manufacturers now offer products made specifically for women, and doctors now know the appropriate conditions for exercise during pregnancy, with the heartening news that sports are healthy for mother and fetus. Coaches, researchers, and physicians are learning how to avoid sports injuries specific to women and their anatomy.

Middle age is often the time when people decide to renew their old sporting interests or to take up a new activity. But those who think their old prowess will return as soon as they step back onto the field are setting the stage for injury and disappointment. Would-be athletes should progress very slowing in becoming fit, giving themselves a year to attain their goals.

Cardiac headaches are recognized by their relationship to exercise; they begin with exertion and are relieved by rest. In the patients that Lipton studied, the headaches disappeared after the patient's heart disease was treated. Treatment ranged from nitroglycerin and other heart disease medications to angioplasty and coronary artery bypass surgery.

........................

# CHAPTER 8

# Treating Orthopedic Injuries

• Breakthroughs have been made in orthopedic treatments for all parts of the body subject to sports injuries.

• The materials and methods being used to repair injuries range from replacing damaged body parts with transplants of your own ligaments, those from cadavers, or synthetics; growing new bone; and intramuscular stimulation, among others.

• The more traditional techniques used to treat injuries and pain, such as heat, cold, RICE, exercise, and physical therapy, remain valuable options—under the right circumstances.

Not long ago, the only remedy for some types of musculoskeletal injuries was an artificial joint. The drawback of course was that such joints could not accommodate vigorous sports play nor could they ever stand the test of time. That made their use questionable in young patients who could anticipate new surgery 10 to 20 years down the line.

Today, the outlook has changed. Scientists can now grow new bone, stimulate hard-to-heal fractures, and repair damaged cartilage with a patient's own cartilage. And there are even more ways to get you back in the game.

# The Shoulder

The shoulder joint is none too stable to begin with, and after some types of injury, surgery may seem to be the only solution. No longer. Doctors now realize that rehabilitative exercise is a viable solution for muscle tears in older, less active patients. And radio-frequency heat probes can now shrink stretched shoulder ligaments to restore stability. When replacement surgery for chronic pain is recommended for severe arthritis or fracture, exercise once again is an integral part of recovery.

## Exercise as Shoulder Therapy

After tearing a shoulder muscle three years ago, Alphonse Weck's shoulder pain was so intense he had to give up playing golf. In fact, he was lucky to be able to brush his teeth. "I could hardly move the left arm at all," he says. "I had almost no side movement at all."

Though Weck suspected that surgery would be the only way to get his shoulder back in shape, he was delighted to find that his doctor's recommendation was actually exercise instead. After six weeks of physical therapy three times a week, the damage had mended.

For shoulder muscle tears in older patients or patients whose shoulders aren't under much stress, a conservative approach of physical therapy may be just the ticket. That's the finding of a Norwegian study of 125 patients with shoulder damage, which found that patients who had physical therapy experienced just as much pain relief and improvement in range of movement as those who had surgery.

"The therapy is a conservative approach," says Seth Newman, physical therapist at the University Medical Center in Tucson, Arizona "If you try it for a couple of months you haven't lost anything at all. There's no reason not to try it."

The downside of the therapy is that it won't work for everyone, particularly those whose shoulder has suffered several tears or who play demanding sports. When it does work, it's 85 percent less costly than surgery and free of dangerous side effects.

# Healing Shoulder Injuries with Heat

The shoulder joint has both the greatest range of motion along with the least stability of any joint in the body, so when ligaments holding the joint in place become lax, the shoulder separates or dislocates. The result is extreme pain and disability. Each year, about 100,000 surgeries are performed to stabilize the shoulder resulting in a three-to-five-inch surgical scar. Cutting through skin, muscle, and tendon, the surgery aims to correct lax shoulder ligaments by trimming and folding loose connective tissue over itself like a pleat and attaching it to the shoulder bone. So invasive is the procedure that it requires extensive hospitalization, plus several months' recuperation. Sadly, even after the surgery, competitive athletes who swim, play volleyball, baseball, or other sports in which the shoulder is considerably challenged only have a 50 percent chance of returning to athletic competition. Shoulder injuries are usually the result of sports, trauma, or birth defects.

Now, surgeons pioneering a new technique called electro-thermal arthroscopy, or ETA, can use radio-frequency heat probes to restore range of motion with less pain, half the recovery time, and greatly increased chances of returning to athletic competition. Through one of two tiny incisions, one in front and one in back of the shoulder, a tiny camera is inserted in the shoulder to examine the overstretched tissue's condition. Heat probes are inserted through the other incision and the radio-frequency energy applied in a sweeping pattern, shrinking the ligaments and stabilizing the shoulder joint.

Not only is it cheaper and less invasive, but it can actually be done in a fraction of the time—under 30 minutes—it takes for the traditional three-hour operation. Best of all, it's actually outpatient surgery, eliminating the need for an extensive period of hospitalization.

"This procedure is especially good news for

competitive athletes and weekend warriors alike, giving them better odds of returning to an active life," says Stephen Liu, M.D., sports medicine orthopedist at UCLA. "Compared to the old way of performing shoulder surgery, ETA is revolutionary. It's like taking a stretched-out pair of blue jeans and throwing them in the dryer to shrink. That's what we can do with the connective tissue surrounding the shoulder joint."

Set at the right temperature to shrink collagen, a connective tissue protein, without damaging it, the effect of the heat probe is startling. It's also considerably safer and less expensive than laser surgery that uses very high heat to cut tissue.

Patients are on their way home in just a few hours postsurgery, says Liu. Instead of nine months of time-consuming rehabilitation, patients like football players Brent Jones, Tim Hanshaw, and Sean Manuel had to be sidelined for only a few games postsurgery.

Furthermore, unlike traditional open surgery, patients lose just 5 to 10 percent of range of motion in the shoulder, and sometimes even less. However, since the surgery is still cutting edge, long-term results are pending.

# Shoulder Replacement

When pain in the ball-and-socket joint of the shoulder becomes chronic and intractable, it may be time to think about getting the joint replaced with an artificial one. Replacing parts of the joint with metal and plastic is proving the solution for some 5,000 people every year. The surgery restores range of motion by resurfacing the shoulder joint, creating a channel in the bone of the upper arm

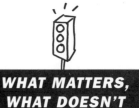

## WHAT MATTERS, WHAT DOESN'T

### What Matters
• Cartilage transplantation as a suitable alternative to joint replacement.

• To repair damaged cartilage with tissue from a donor.

• Opting for proven procedures that have clinical studies showing how techniques stand up over time.

### What Doesn't
• Getting the newest experimental technique or invention.

• Living with pain and postponing surgery until there's no other option.

and filling it with a metal ball on a stem to replace damaged bone. No pain occurs at the joint since the materials don't have nerve fibers. Used to treat shoulders crippled by arthritis or those fractured by severe trauma, an important component of the cure is rehabilitation exercises to restore fuller range of motion.

## Repairing Rotator Cuff Tears

Swimmers, racquet-sports players, and basketball players, whose sports demand extensive overhead movement, are at risk for tears in the shoulder's rotator cuff. Now a more conservative surgery in which the coracoacromial ligament under the collarbone is left in place, rather than removed as it is in more in traditional surgery, appears to get patients back in action faster and less painfully.

At Georgetown University, orthopedists operated on 86 patients to mend the tears, leaving the coracoacromial ligament in place. Just under 85 percent of those in the study reported little pain, only minor decrease in range of motion, and few other side effects, and were able to begin rehabbing the shoulder within a few days postsurgery. By three months, many were already able to start playing sports again! Ninety-three percent of patients reported satisfaction with the procedure.

## The Elbow

Elbows become injured as a result of overuse. Sometimes the "cure" only prolongs the pain and disability syndrome. Now there's a new theory as to the real reason injuries like tennis elbow occur and how to treat them!

# Cortisone and RICE: NO!

You're getting the wrong treatment if your doctor wants to remedy tennis elbow symptoms with cortisone injections. According to Robert P. Nirschle, M.D., author of *Arm Care,* both cortisone and RICE are the wrong treatments. What's really behind the pain is what he calls "a heart attack of the tendon" resulting in blockage of blood vessels or breakdown of the protein in the tendon. He thinks a better name for the condition is tendonosis, rather than tendinitis.

Therapy for a blocked tendon is to create new blood vessels and protein, not to relieve inflammation. Nirschle says trying to treat the condition as an inflammation is off base because there are no inflammatory cells in the tissue to treat.

## A Patch to Heal Sports Pain

When you've injured yourself playing sports, you want pain relief fast. Pills will eventually do the trick, but first they have to navigate the body's anatomy, arriving at long last at their destination. With the new pain patch, all you do is slap it on where it hurts. No trying not to forget to take your pain medication. Widely available in Europe, the patch is still in clinical trials in the United States, but FDA approval is expected soon. For now, it's being tested only for sports injuries relief. Down the road, there will be applications to arthritis and muscle aches.

# Exercise: Yes!

The key to accomplishing all this blood-vessel and protein creation is exercise. Because tennis elbow is a complex condition involving dysfunction in muscles throughout the arm, that means building up muscles from the rotator cuff to the wrist. Most of the exercises he recommends are familiar—wrist curls, shoulder shrugs, biceps curls.

Having a strong, well-conditioned musculoskeletal structure as a base on which to build sports prowess and treat pain is one of the most important tenets of sports medicine. Nirschle's recommended treatment may be just the ticket for those athletes willing to work at rehab rather than just treating tennis elbow with a skin prick.

# Hips

Because of the tremendous load that's placed on the hips, fractures can be devastating, even crippling. But science has come a long way in resolving those fears, first with artificial joints, then with processes that stimulate the growth of new bone so that young, active people have a better alternative than hip replacement.

## Hip Replacement

In 1998 more than 50,000 people under age 50 received total hip replacements. Heralded as the best method to replace cartilage loss in the knees or hips of young patients who'd suffered trauma or disease, doctors now realize that artificial joint replacement is not well suited for younger, more active patients. Though hip replacement makes patients mobile, the joints themselves invariably need replacement one or more times again during their lives.

# Bone Morphogenetic Protein

Today, orthopedic researchers at the University of California, Los Angeles have developed a new technique to treat bone death in human hips that could prevent the need for a total replacement. Each year, about 20,000 new cases of the condition are diagnosed. Though the jury is still out on why the blood supply becomes cut off, researchers have traced the condition to three factors—hip trauma, alcoholism, or steroid drug use. Called osteoregeneration, the procedure implants a capsule filled with bone morphogenetic protein (BMP) to stimulate the body to grow more bone.

Just what is bone death? "It occurs when the blood supply to the head of the femur bone dies," explains Jay Lieberman, M.S., assistant professor of orthopedic surgery at UCLA and the originator of the osteoregeneration procedure. "The femoral head is the knobby end of the thighbone that fits into the hip socket."

The key to making the procedure successful is to do the surgery early before too much bone dies. Otherwise, the femoral head will collapse under the weight of the hip joint.

The use of BMP is new. Prior to its development, UCLA surgeons performed core decompression, involving the drilling of a hole into the femoral head to remove the dead bone. Now,

**SMART MOVE**

"Thanks to osteoregeneration with bone morphogenetic protein (BMP), people who once couldn't walk across a room without pain are now back to hiking, golfing, and fully active lives," explains Jay Lieberman, M.S., assistant professor of orthopedic surgery at UCLA, who originated the procedure. "Of course, those who stand the best chance of doing well with the procedure are youngish [under 60], active, and in good health with limited bone loss in the hip."

• Ultrasound waves—like those used to examine a fetus—stimulate fractured bone to heal faster.

• Ultrasound use can decrease the time it takes for new bone to generate by approximately 40 percent.

• By saving healing time, the procedure saves money in lost wages and reduces the need for additional surgery.

Lieberman inserts a BMP implant into the cavity, followed by an implant of purified human bone also containing BMP to lend structural support to the joint during healing.

So far, Lieberman has done about a dozen cases. Patients report good to excellent relief in pain. Since the procedure is still in clinical trials, injured recreational athletes might want to consider other methods of correcting bone death in the hip:

• To relieve pressure on the femoral head in the earliest stages of osteonecrosis, surgeons drill into the bone, restoring blood flow and encouraging growth of new bone.

• For patients with minimal bone damage to the area, surgeons can perform an osteotomy in which the femoral head is rotated. That way, weight-bearing is left to the healthy part of the bone.

# Bone Grafting

At the University of Pittsburgh, Duke University, Mount Sinai Hospital in Toronto, and Case Western Reserve University in Cleveland, young, active people have still another option—grafts of bone from other parts of the body. In these grafts, dead bone is replaced by transplanted living bone and blood vessels are reattached so that the bone can grow. This procedure has been successful in four out of five of the surgeries performed at the University of Pittsburgh Medical Center, and those who have the surgery have even done well enough to return to playing golf.

## Treating Severe Bruises

Laser treatment is proving an alternative to physical rehabilitation in treating severe bruises.

Optical energy at low levels reaches deep into tissue to stimulate healing. Called the Theralase Laser System, the new technology is being studied in patients with a variety of sports injuries and chronic pain. Results show a faster decrease in pain and healing time, with faster improvement in flexibility and range of motion. The treatment itself is not painful; the only sensation that patients feel is heat.

"We're seeing 85 to 90 percent positive results using the Theralase Laser to treat patients with sprains, tendinitis, osteoarthritis, and other injuries," Lyndi Robinson, M.S., physical therapist at Doctors Hospital in Dallas told *Medical Breakthroughs* (www.ivanhoe.com). "Patients are responding much more quickly."

# Pelvic Osteotomy

Young to middle-aged adults from their 30s to 50s who face the possibility of hip replacement surgery because of premature onset of arthritis now have a new and better option. Called periacetabular pelvic osteotomy, the procedure produces good pain relief and increased mobility. It's relatively new, having been introduced about a decade ago.

"Until this was developed, there was no completely satisfactory therapy for younger adults with hip arthritis caused by an underdevelopment of the hip," explains Richard F. Santore, M.D., clinical professor of orthopedics with the University of California San Diego (UCSD) School of Medicine and chief of orthopedics service at UCSD's Thornton Hospital. "In young patients, artificial replacements are not ideal as they can wear out in three to five years. Pelvic osteotomy, on the other hand, may postpone the need for an artificial hip for 20 years or more."

In pelvic osteotomy, surgeons separate the hip joint from the pelvis, rotate it to a normal position and bolt it into place. This protects the joint from further deterioration so that Santore says patients are walking normally within three months post-surgery. No casts or braces are needed.

# The Back

Back injuries and back pain send more people to the doctor than almost any other injury or illness. Too often the advice is an invasive surgery that requires lengthy recuperation, and when it's over, patients are very frequently in no better shape than before the procedure. New breakthroughs in treating back injuries promise to end this frustrating scenario.

## Repairing Herniated Disks

In about the same time it takes to change the oil in your car, an athlete with a herniated disk displaced from its position between the vertebrae can get it repaired. At Sinai Hospital of Baltimore, orthopedic surgeon Mark Rosenthal, M.D., is using microsurgery to remove the degenerated part of the herniated disk, relieving pressure on the nerves and related numbness and pain. The procedure can also treat bone spurs that are often the by-product of degenerating disks.

The tiny one-inch incision through which the surgery is accomplished means that muscles are left intact so that recuperation is fast. Whereas patients undergoing the standard surgical procedure for herniated disks are hospitalized for almost a week, those that have the hour-long microdiskectomy are discharged the same day.

"Getting patients out of bed immediately following surgery prevents the joint stiffness and weakness that occurs with bed rest," says Rosenthal. "In about six weeks most patients are able to get back to just about every activity they used to do before."

## Intramuscular Stimulation: Alternative to Disk Surgery

Doctors in the electrodiagnosis laboratory at the University of Pennsylvania Medical Center have devised a new pain-relief strategy for chronic back pain due to injured nerves and degenerating structures in the spine. It's also useful in alleviating nerve-related pain elsewhere in the body. Called Automated Twitch-Obtaining Intramuscular Stimulation (ATOIMS), it employs a battery-operated automated device that shoots three needles in seconds into muscles on the receiving end of the pain message line.

"ATOIMS is clinically proven to provide relief for soft-tissue pain that originates in the muscles, tendons, ligaments, and the areas surrounding bones," says Jennifer Chu, M.D., who is director of the lab. "The procedure involves inserting fine Teflon pins deep into the muscle and motor endplate zones (the nerves that stimulate muscles to

**STREET SMARTS**

Accountant Jim Fetterman, 28, struggled with groin and back pain for seven years. In January 1998, Jim began ATOIMS treatment. A weight trainer and avid runner, Jim had developed spinal stenosis and a male pelvic pain condition. "I was at the point where I was living with pain—unable to work out, having a hard time working or performing any of my regular activities."

After six months, Jim was able to walk again without pain. "Today, I still can't lift heavy weights, but I can walk two to four miles a day on the treadmill without pain," he says. "I would never be able to do that without the treatment." Jim has been able to cut back on treatment sessions, and will continue to reduce his treatment schedule until he has no need at all.

"I jogged, trekked, and played a lot of real hard tennis," says Jacque Gary, 67. That kind of pounding put more stress on the knee cartilage than it could take, causing it to thin and depleting fluid in the knee that helps cushion shock. "The result was pain—and a lot of it," she says. In a desperate attempt to remain active and put off a knee replacement as long as possible, she signed up for a series of Synvisc injections. "I'm a real busy person and don't like to be slowed down," she says of her decision.

contract and produce movement) where irritated nerve fibers and shortened muscle fibers causing pain are found. Inserting pins into these trigger points causes the muscle fibers to automatically twitch, increasing blood flow to the site. Simultaneously, the twitching interrupts the shortening of the muscle fibers by exercising them, permitting the fibers to relax so that self-healing can begin."

The first device of its kind, ATOIMS marries acupuncture with high-tech. It's best designed for treating traumatic conditions—athletic injuries, whiplash, unprotected falls, and lifting injuries—as well as aging-related problems. Such injuries precipitate a domino effect as the irritated nerve roots signal the muscles to shorten and spasm, causing blood vessels and nerves to compress and pull on the tendons, bones, joints, and ligaments. The result is discomfort and pain.

ATOIMS has no side effects, causes no nerve damage, and is more precise than acupuncture. It targets trigger points where nerve fibers meet muscle fibers that supply feedback to the spinal cord. It was developed to penetrate the skin more rapidly, allowing the pin to be injected and retracted three times in the same position.

# The Knee

Athletes with chronic knee pain due to osteoarthritis (which affects almost 14 million Americans) now have dramatic help in relieving the pain and stiffness that usually follows exercise.

# Alternatives to Total Knee Replacement

## Synvisc

A series of three injections a week for three weeks of a new medication called Synvisc cushions the surfaces inside the knee, relieving pain for up to 18 months. This therapy is helpful for patients over 40 who haven't responded to traditional treatments such as over-the-counter anti-inflammatory medications, cortisone injections, exercise, or physical therapy and whose only other option is a total knee replacement.

## Hedrocel

In young patients like Greta Lacy, 26, the danger of knee replacement surgery is that the implanted joint will loosen, leading to yet another operation. To avoid that scenario, Audrey Tsao, M.D., associate professor of orthopedic surgery at the University of Mississippi Medical Center, decided to use Hedrocel, a new orthopedic implant material manufactured by Implex. It's composed of 98 percent tantalum, a noncorrosive, moldable metal used in other prosthetic devices.

"What's so unique about this new material is it allows bones and tissue to grow through and around it," says Tsao. "The design reduces wear and tear on the implant and makes surgical implantation easier and faster."

Tsao designs implants for her patients and helped custom fit a knee for Lacy. Designing the knee to fit took about a year to complete, but surgery took just a day.

**STREET SMARTS**

Greta Lacey, 26, thought she'd never walk again after a 1994 car accident. "My leg was pinned in the car for six hours," she says. "Circulation to the bottom half of the leg was cut, and my knee was crushed. Doctors told me I had two choices—a rod implanted in my leg that wouldn't allow me to bend my knee or amputation." Instead, at the University of Mississippi Medical Center, she had a new knee joint fashioned from an innovative material called Hedrocel. "Doctors say this could well last me a lifetime!"

# Anterior Cruciate Ligament (ACL) Transplant

Because the anterior cruciate ligament—located in the center of the knee joint, to help support and stabilize the knee—prevents excessive forward motion of the leg, an ACL rupture invariably once meant the end of an athlete's career. That's what gymnast and Olympic gold medalist Bart Conner was looking at after injuring two knee ligaments including the ACL. Lucky for Conner, doctors were able to transplant a knee tendon from a cadaver, putting the athlete back on track.

Treated in 1986 by Lonnie Paulos, M.D., then orthopedic surgeon at the Orthopedic Specialty Hospital in Salt Lake City, the new procedure involved transplanting a fresh frozen patellar tendon from a cadaver into Conner's knee. Thanks to the transplant, Conner was actually able to return to professional play six months later.

"The track record for this procedure has been outstanding with about 95 percent of patients recovering almost completely," says Paulos. "In the first five to six years following surgery, these transplants increase stability, muscle strength, and mobility, and decrease pain. The procedure allows the surgeon to create a stronger new ligament by using transplanted tissue instead of weakening the patient's own tendons through an autograft (transplant of a patient's own tendon)."

"We have critically analyzed the variables that allowed patients to return to athletic activities," said Don Shelbourne, M.D., team physician for the Indianapolis Colts, who has analyzed results of surgery to repair the anterior cruciate ligament (ACL) on 1,057 patients. "Patients had to have sufficient strength to run, pivot, and jump. In order to do so, we had to make sure that they had good strength in their quadriceps muscle and minimized swelling in the knee. We concluded that most patients who followed an accelerated rehabilitation program returned to full function quickly and exhibited positive long-term results."

## Knee Plugs

If you injure your articular cartilage on the end of the knee bones, you'll feel sharp pain on both sides of the knee and you won't be able to walk. Forget having the injury heal on its own; there's just not enough blood supply to the area. If you ignore it, you'll develop arthritis and the knee's ability to maneuver will deteriorate. Normally, such injuries are corrected by surgically removing the damaged cartilage. But Freddie Fu, M.D., orthopedic surgeon at the University of Pittsburgh Medical Center in Pennsylvania, has pioneered a novel new procedure in which he transplants healthy living cartilage from the edge of the knee into the damaged spot. After surgery, it takes about one to two months to get the knees ready to bear weight. The next step is physical rehabilitation.

In use in Europe for several years, this procedure has only recently been introduced to the United States.

## Growing New Knees

There's little that will put an athlete out of commission faster than a knee injury. Each year, about

**F.Y.I.**

According to a 1997 study involving 1,057 patients (presented to the American Orthopaedic Society for Sports Medicine), from 1990 to 1997, 76 percent of patients undergoing reconstruction of their anterior cruciate ligament (ACL) were back playing sports within two months postsurgery.

Most were competing at full capacity by six months.

900,000 knee cartilage injuries occur from sports and other traumas. Up until recently, most sufferers could look forward to the eventual and almost inevitable stint on the operating table for an artificial knee.

No longer. Now people with certain types of damaged cartilage on the thighbone part of the knee have a new option—repairing the damage with their own cultured cartilage. Best of all, the procedure works very well in people who engage in active sports or who have complex injuries.

The name of the therapy is Carticel, and it is made by Genzyme Tissue Repair. It's designed to replace surgery for knee joints that can no longer function normally because of damage to the articular cartilage, a thin layer of tough tissue covering the ends of bones where they connect in the joint. When the cartilage is injured, pain, limited range of motion, and even osteoarthirits can develop. In such cases, the body won't heal itself because this cartilage won't regrow. Limited blood supply to the structure also restricts its ability to heal.

Before Carticel, repairing the cartilage involved surgery to smooth out the damage, plus a number of techniques to create fibrous or scar tissue to ensure a smooth gliding surface needed for the joint to function.

"The cartilage we're replacing with the Carticel transplant is called the hyaline cartilage," Mark Hollmann, orthopedic surgeon and sports medicine physician at the Columbia Deland Surgery Center in Deland, Florida, said in *Carticel: Growing New Knees* (published online by Galen Health Care). "It covers the end of the bone and looks like the white shiny stuff in the end of a chicken bone. In the past, when that was damaged or injured, the only thing we could really do was to shave it with an arthroscope and hope that what's called fiber cartilage or scar type of cartilage would form."

Though the scar tissue does help by covering the joint surface, it isn't as strong and long-lasting as normal cartilage, especially for active people who enjoy sports. Pain often returns so that patients must either undergo repeat surgery, even a total joint replacement with an artificial knee, or simply decide to accept the pain and limitations on mobility.

Those 200,000 who opt for knee replacement each year must also contend with the possibility that it will have to be repeated 10 to 15 years down the line, making it a not very viable option for those under age 50.

Enter Carticel. After a surgeon takes a biopsy of healthy cartilage, millions of new cells are grown, then implanted into the knee later. During the operation, damaged tissue is removed, the cells implanted and covered by a small piece of the periosteum taken from the skin covering a bone. As the cultured cells multiply, they integrate with surrounding cartilage to grow new bone. Since the surgery involves implanting the patient's own cells, there's no possibility of tissue rejection. Within a year postsurgery, many patients are back living normal lives.

In March 1998, a long-term 5- and 10-year study of patients in whom the procedure had been done was completed. It revealed just how well Carticel works. Ninety-six percent of those who had good to excellent results two years after the surgery were still doing well a decade later.

Orthopedic surgeons report that 85 percent of patients treated with Carticel showed improvement in key areas—clinician and patient evaluations of overall knee condition, patient reports of

## STREET SMARTS

"One month after arthroscopic surgery to repair cartilage in my knee, it was making the same popping and catching and grinding stuff again," says Jay Wallace. "A few months after I had the Carticel implant, I'm back on my bike and expect to go in-line skating. I feel great, excellent. I feel like it's going to be just like nothing ever happened to me."

symptoms such as pain and swelling, and knee examination results.

Ninety percent of all patients treated worldwide as of November 1998 reported no complications, with just 5 percent reporting adverse problems at least possibly related to Carticel.

Since its implementation, 91 percent of patients have reported no additional surgical procedures following Carticel implantation; the operations that were done were minor and done with an arthroscope.

Carticel is outstandingly successful with young people between the ages of 15 and 55. Prior to the Carticel implant, 71 percent of the patients had undergone at least one procedure on the treated knee in the previous five years, and 59 percent were treated surgically for articular injuries.

## New Brace Helps Sports Participation

A specially designed and fitted brace may help people with certain knee problems participate in sports and fitness activities again, says the American Orthopaedic Society for Sports Medicine. Called an "unloader brace," it's designed to "relieve pressure from the inner side of the knee caused by mild degenerative diseases like osteoarthirits," says Tom Wickiewicz, M.D., chief of the sports medicine and shoulder service at the Hospital for Special Surgery in New York. The brace works by applying pressure and redistributing the load or force a person puts on their knee when walking or running. It can also help alleviate the pain of symptomatic knock-kneedness or bowleggedness. It's available by prescription from an orthopedic surgeon.

"Most patients find that they are able to be much more active wearing this brace because they aren't held back by pain," says Wickiewicz.

Carticel is the only such product approved by the Food and Drug Administration.

## Grafting for Young Knees

Another alternative for young adults who need damaged cartilage in their knees and ankles repaired is fresh osteochondral allografting or cartilage transplantation. In this procedure, only damaged tissue and a small section of connecting bone is removed and replaced with healthy donor tissue and bone that the orthopedic surgeon has shaped to an exact fit. Within a few months, the donor material knits into the patient's own, forming a strong and stable bond able to withstand the stress of an athletic lifestyle.

# The Hand and Wrist

Together, the hand and wrist comprise more bones, muscles, and ligaments than are found in any other single region of the body. Sports as well as work and day-to-day activities can be the culprit for a sidelining injury But the options of treating hand and wrist pain are more varied than ever.

## Relief from Carpal Tunnel Syndrome (CTS)

About 1 in 10 people who perform repetitive movements with their hands (like typists and computer operators, even hair dressers) can develop

### STREET SMARTS

When Daniel Mashburn was 13, he seriously injured his knee in a water-skiing accident. He didn't realize the extent of the damage and, despite some pain, he continued surfing, biking, and water skiing. "Over the years my knee continued to deteriorate, and the pain ultimately got so bad I could barely walk," says Mashburn, now 39 and a marketing consultant. "I was facing a total knee replacement until I met Dr. Bugbee." Four years ago Mashburn underwent osteochondral allografting for his knee at the UCSD Medical School. Today he's back at the gym three or four times a week, working with weights, doing aerobics, and taking 14-mile bicycle rides two to five times a week. "I can do all the things I love!" he says.

## THE BOTTOM LINE

Treatment options available today range from radio-frequency heat probes that shrink tendons and stabilize joints, to man-made replacement joints, to a pain patch capable of delivering quick relief directly to the site of an injury. In place of undergoing a total hip or knee replacement is bone morphogenetic protein (BMP) implants, which stimulate growth of new bone. Another alternative is to transplant bone from other parts of the body, along with its blood supply, to encourage new bone growth. New alternatives are being explored every day, and research and development have gone far to ensure that active individuals have a range of options to help them deal with pain and injury.

chronic wrist pain, numbness, tingling, and radiating pain through the upper arm due to a compressed nerve. Severe cases require surgery, but a third of those who undergo the procedure find themselves back in the operating room because of postoperative scar tissue buildup. The result is more painful pressure on the nerve so that patients find themselves back where they started. Now, a new procedure in which a vein is removed from the lower leg and wrapped around the nerve appears to prevent new scar tissue from forming around the nerve. Eighty percent of the small sampling of patients who have undergone the procedure have had excellent to good long-term results.

# On the Horizon . . .

A year from now, surgeons expect to cure hard-to-heal bone fractures through a process of genetic engineering accomplished via bone marrow aspiration. Stem cells (the parent cells from which all organs in the body are produced) removed from the patient receive genes that stimulate production of growth-inducing proteins, then they're reimplanted. Enough new bone grows to heal the injury.

Sound like science fiction? For people who suffer the damage and loss of bones, joints, tissues, and cartilage due to disease, injury, age, and even periodontal disease, techniques like these often eliminate the need for amputation, artificial implants, and disability.

It's never been easier to treat orthopedic injuries and get athletes back into play.

# Index

# Books in the
# Smart Guide™ series

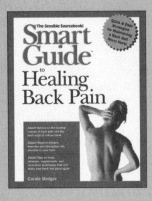

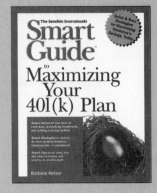

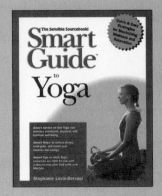

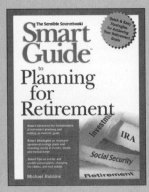

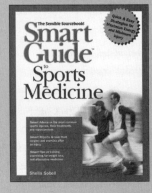

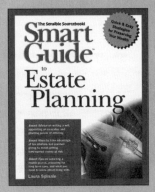